MATTER OF MIND

MATTER
OF
MIND

A Neurologist's View of Brain-Behavior Relationships

Kenneth M. Heilman, M.D.

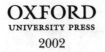

OXFORD
UNIVERSITY PRESS
2002

OXFORD
UNIVERSITY PRESS

Oxford   New York
Auckland   Bangkok   Buenos Aires   Cape Town   Chennai
Dar es Salaam   Delhi   Hong Kong   Istanbul   Karachi   Kolkata
Kuala Lumpur   Madrid   Melbourne   Mexico City   Mumbai   Nairobi
São Paulo   Shanghai   Singapore   Taipei   Tokyo   Toronto

and an associated company in Berlin

Copyright © 2002 by Oxford University Press, Inc.

Published by Oxford University Press Inc.
198 Madison Avenue, New York, New York 10016
http://www.oup-usa.org
1-800-334-4249

Oxford is a registered trademark of Oxford University Press.

Library of Congress Cataloging-in-Publication Data
Heilman, Kenneth M., 1938–
Matter of mind: a neurologist's view of brain-behavior relationships / Kenneth M. Heilman.
p. : cm.
Includes bibliographical references and index.
ISBN 0-19-514490-2
1. Higher nervous activity.   2. Neuropsychology.   3. Neuropsychiatry.
4. Neurobehavioral disorders.   I. Title.
[DNLM: 1. Brain Diseases–physiopathology.   2. Behavior-physiology.
3. Behavioral Symptoms–physiopathology.
4. Brain-physiology.   5. Mental Processes–physiology.
WL 348 H466m 2002]
QP395 .H45 2002
616.8—dc21
2001036399

1 3 5 7 9 8 6 4 2

Printed in the United States of America
on acid-free paper

This book is dedicated to
my immediate family:
Rosalind,
Samuel,
Fred,
Patricia,
David,
Nicole,
Chip,
Eden,
and Brooke

PREFACE

The mind is the product of the brain's activities, and the brain's activities depend on its organization. Just over 100 years ago Santiago Ramón y Cajal revealed that the brain is composed of individual cells, most of which are called *neurons*. The human brain weighs only about 3 pounds, but it is estimated to contain more than 10 billion neurons. Most of these cells are found in the cerebral cortex, the covering mantle of the brain. In this 3-mm-thick structure there are six layers of neurons. At the turn of the twentieth century, Korbinian Brodmann noticed that different anatomical areas of the cerebral cortex had different neuronal configurations. These differences depend on how the neurons in the areas are connected to other parts of the brain. Neurons in the brain gather information from the outside world and from our body. They send information to and receive information from other nerve cells. Thus, the billions of neurons have trillions of connections with each other. Knowledge is stored in the brain by the type and strength of connections between these neurons. Brain neurons also send instructions to the body that control our actions.

Mental faculties can be divided into at least eight major categories or domains: cognition (thinking or the processing of stored knowledge), emotion, attention, memory, motor skills, self awareness (or consciousness), perception, and conation (or drive). Each of these domains has multiple subcategories. For example, speech, reading, and writing are all subcategories of cognition. While this book discusses each of the major categories, a detailed discussion of all the subcategories is beyond its scope.

There are many ways to study the brain. Although anatomical and physiological studies can help us understand the substrates of behavior, most of what we have learned about how the brain mediates behavior comes from experiments of nature in which focal brain injuries induced by diseases such as stroke produce behavioral changes. This book focuses on what the *lesion* method has taught us about how the brain works. After an area of the brain (e.g., the left frontal lobe) is injured, patients may lose the ability to perform a certain type of behavior (e.g., speak). Damage in another area of the brain (e.g., the left occipital lobe) may cause a different deficit (e.g., reading disability). Although the lesion method has proven to be very useful in helping us understand brain functions, it depends on the assumption that when a function is lost due to brain damage, the damaged area is critical for performing the function. Because other areas of the brain might be able to assume the functions of the damaged area, this assumption is not always correct. To help document how specific areas of the brain work, it is important to obtain converging evidence from a variety of other approaches such as electrophysiological recording and functional imaging.

For patients and their families, brain damage is often a tragic event that causes disability and suffering, but the behavioral studies we perform do not hurt these patients. When I first started to study patients, I was concerned about bothering them or making them feel depressed because I was testing their deficits. Of course, before testing patients we obtain their consent, explain that our studies probably will not help them, and tell them that our primary purpose is to learn how the brain works. We have found that most people are genuinely altruistic. After thanking our patients and their families for helping us carry out this neurobehavioral research, I have often heard them say that they hope the research will help someone else and that participating in it has made them feel better. In addition, many of the tests we perform do enable patients to better understand the nature of their deficits, and this understanding may help them develop alternative strategies for coping with their disabilities. We are also beginning to learn that cognitive stimulation may aid recovery and that testing is a form of cognitive stimulation. This book will describe many of the patients my colleagues and I have examined, tested, and studied. To protect their privacy, I've changed their names, altered situations, and added fictional touches.

I have been studying the brain for more than 35 years. As a physician, I hoped that these studies would help improve the care of patients with diseases of the brain, but I also wanted to know how nature's greatest masterpiece works. It is my hope that people who are curious about how the brain works will enjoy reading about what we and others have learned. Unlike standard texts, this book does not contain references, but for those who want more information I have listed some suggested readings at the end of each chapter.

I would like to thank the patients who served as subjects for our studies. They and their families have been generous with their time and energy. They have also been very kind to our technicians, students, residents, and fellows. In addition, many of them have encouraged our young investigators, and this has been important in helping many of these trainees launch productive research careers.

Over the past thirty years many wonderful people have come to Gainesville to work with me. Few things have brought me as much joy or as many rewards as teaching and learning from these people. In this book I mention many of my current and former students, as well as other colleagues. Although I could not give credit to everyone, they all have my gratitude. I would also like to thank Jeff House at Oxford University Press, who helped me shape this book.

Gainesville, Florida   K.M.H.

CONTENTS

MATTER OF MIND

CHAPTER

1

INTRODUCTION

Philosophy and religion have profound influences on science, but they are often adverse. Though Aristotle had a tremendous impact on the development of Western thought, he believed that the mind and thinking had no relationship to the body, including the brain. The idea that the mind is separate from the brain is called *dualism*. Even today there are those who adhere to a dualistic philosophy. It is not my purpose to engage in this debate, but rather simply to state that accepting dualism would preclude studying the relationships between the brain and mental functions such as language, memory, perception, attention, conation, and self-awareness. In contrast to Aristotle, Hippocrates, the Greek physician and founder of Western medicine, thought that the brain was the organ of intellect. Like Hippocrates, we know that some diseases of the brain such as stroke may cause sudden and dramatic changes in behavior and thought. We also know that other diseases such as Alzheimer disease cause progressive degradation of the mind.

One way of approaching the study of brain–behavior relationships is to use a model system borrowed from another field. Herophilus, for instance, may have used hydraulic engineering principles
to explain brain function. Cerebral spinal fluid (CSF) flows around
the brain and is stored within intracerebral cavities called *ventricles*.
It travels through tunnels called *aqueducts*, and between the skull and
brain it is stored in cavities called *cisterns*. About 300 B.C.E., Herophilus posited that the flow patterns of CSF are responsible for
thought and that the brain substance is the supporting infrastructure
of this fluid system. About 100 years later, Galen, who practiced in
the ancient city of Pergamum (now Bergama, Turkey), made the
counterproposal that it is not the flow of CSF that is important for
thought and knowledge but rather the brain substance. Although we
cannot be certain why Herophilus believed that the brain's fluid
system is responsible for thought, it obviously involved his dependence upon analogy or metaphor. In the late classical Greek and
early Roman periods, one of the major engineering advances was
hydraulics, including the movement of fresh water and fluid wastes.
Even today we can visit ancient Roman aqueducts and cisterns. Using
engineering principles to model brain function has a long history
and continues today as many investigators borrow ideas from computer engineering and some people believe that the brain is little
more than a biological digital computer.

As mentioned in the preface the major active unit in the brain
is the nerve cell, or neuron. There are billions of neurons in the
human brain, and each one communicates directly and indirectly
with hundreds or thousands of other nerve cells. Some of these connections (*synapses*) may be strong and others weak. Some are excitatory and others inhibitory. With learning, these connections can
change, and the storage of information depends upon the connec-
tivity and excitability of neuronal ensembles. Computers are able to
model many of the brain's cognitive systems, and these models allow
neuroscientists to ask new questions. Neuroscientists, however,
should keep in mind the blunder made by Herophilus. We must
remember that while engineering models may help generate new
hypotheses about brain function, these hypotheses must be tested in
biological systems.

During the Middle Ages it was illegal to perform postmortem
studies, but curious people like Vesalius violated this law by studying
anatomy in corpses. The understanding of function is aided by the

understanding of structure, and Vesalius wrote extensively about the anatomy of the brain. The next major advance in understanding brain–behavior relationships did not occur until the seventeenth century, when Descartes became interested in the pineal gland. This is the only intracranial structure that is unpaired. In addition, it is located near the geographic center of the brain. Based on its anatomical location, Descartes proposed that the pineal gland was the seat of the soul because all things must enter or emanate from the soul and its central location made the pineal gland well positioned for this function. Today we know that the pineal gland is an endocrine gland that produces melatonin, thought to be important in sleep. Although Descartes was incorrect about the function of the pineal gland, his idea that a structure of the brain is important in carrying out a specific function and that this function depends on this structure's anatomy were important new constructs.

In the eighteenth century, Franz Gall also put forth a more elaborate view of the localization of brain functions. He thought that intellect was mediated by the two cerebral hemispheres, united by the corpus callosum, and that the brain stem was important for controlling vital functions such as respiration. He also proposed that the different human faculties mediated by the brain are located in different areas of the cerebral cortex. During development, the growth and shape of the skull depend upon growth of the brain. According to Gall if certain brain functions are mediated by specific anatomical areas (a view now termed *modularity*), then the more brain tissue devoted to these functions, the better they would be performed. Since the size of the brain region devoted to a function influences the shape of the skull overlying this area, one should be able to measure a person's ability to perform different functions by measuring portions of her or his skull. These theories led to the pseudoscience of phrenology and its many unfounded claims about skull shapes and mental abilities. These claims were not substantiated by scientific evidence. The widespread practice of phrenology quickly ended when most of its claims were found to be incorrect. Nonetheless, Gall's concepts of anatomical localization and functional modularity were important in the development of cognitive neuroscience.

Anthropologists have taken a strong interest in skull measurements. In the mid-nineteenth century Paul Broca, a French physician and anthropologist, heard a lecture by one of Gall's students, who noted that fluent speakers have prominent foreheads and suggested that the facility of speech is mediated by the frontal lobes of the brain. At the time, there was a diabetic man on Broca's hospital service who was suffering with gangrene. Years earlier, the man had had a stroke and lost the faculty of speech. Unfortunately, in the nineteenth century there were no antibiotics to treat gangrene, and the man died. Postmortem examination revealed a predominantly left frontal lesion. Broca subsequently described eight patients who were right-handed and who had lost their speech from damage to the left hemisphere. Broca's observations supported Gall's postulate of localized function and led to what Thomas Kuhn, in his book *The Structure of Scientific Revolutions*, calls a *paradigmatic shift*—the start of a new science. Today this science takes many forms, including neuropsychology, behavioral neurology, behavioral neuroscience, and cognitive neuroscience.

About 10 years after Broca published his findings, the German neurologist Carl Wernicke reported a patient who could speak fluently but could not comprehend speech. In addition to describing a new language disorder, Wernicke made two important conceptual advances. First, he demonstrated a double dissociation. In order to show that an anatomical area of the brain is critical for mediating a specific function (e.g., fluent speech), one must demonstrate that with injury to this area this function is lost but another function (e.g., speech comprehension) is preserved. Broca had already demonstrated this single dissociation. To establish modularity fully, however, a double dissociation is needed: one has to demonstrate that when one area is damaged (e.g., the left frontal lobe), one function is lost (e.g., speech fluency) but another is preserved (e.g., speech comprehension), and when a different brain area is damaged, the function lost with the prior lesion (e.g., fluency) is preserved but the function preserved with the first lesion (e.g., speech comprehension) is now lost. Wernicke reported a patient who had fluent speech but poor speech comprehension. This patient had a left posterior hemisphere lesion that was anatomically distinct from the anterior lesion that Broca reported to be associated with a nonfluent aphasia. Wernicke's patient together with Broca's patient met the double dissociation criterion for localized function or modularity.

Wernicke also initiated the development of information-processing models. His clinical observations suggested that the left posterior area of the brain contains the auditory memories of how words sound, and that normally this posterior area is able to send this word sound information to the anterior area, which Broca had found to be important in programming the movements needed to speak. From this new information-processing model one could make new predictions. For example, if these two regions were intact but disconnected by damage to the pathway that connects them, a patient should be fluent and able to comprehend, but when speaking, naming, or repeating, the patient would use the wrong speech sounds because the posterior area that contains the memories of word sounds could not provide the anterior area with this information. Subsequently, this type of disorder, predicted by Wernicke's information-processing model, was described and is called *conduction aphasia.*

Information-processing models help us understand how the brain works and enable us to ask further questions about brain functions. They presume that the brain is modular and that there is both serial and parallel processing. Recent studies using strong magnets to detect small brain currents (magnetoencephalography) have permitted neuroscientists to measure the time that elapses between stimulus presentation and activation of cortical anatomical areas. These studies demonstrate that serial processing, as predicted by information-processing models, does occur.

About 200 years after Gall postulated brain specialization (modularity), size–function relationships (bigger is better), and asymmetries of skull growth accompanying specialization, Norman Geschwind demonstrated that the posterior area of the brain that stores memories of words' sounds (Wernicke's area) is larger in the left (language-dominant) hemisphere than in the right hemisphere. Using computed tomography (CT) scans, Marjorie LaMay later showed that the portion of skull covering this specialized language area bulges out more on the left side than on the right. By measuring the skull on CT scans, neurologists can predict which hemisphere is dominant for mediating speech, thereby supporting Gall's original hypothesis, but they cannot predict personality traits, as claimed by the phrenologists.

Broca's and Wernicke's seminal studies led to the golden age of neuropsychology that lasted until the First World War. Many of the disorders described in this book were first reported during that period, but after the war the localizationist–connectionist approach of Paul Broca, Wernicke, and their colleagues was abandoned. The reason for this demise is not entirely clear, but there were probably two

major factors: poor science and a change in the political–philosoph-
ical zeitgeist. After the First World War, the continental European
powers such as Germany and France lost much of their power and
influence on Western thought. In contrast, the English-speaking
countries such as the United States and the United Kingdom flour-
ished. The American and British social and political systems were
strongly influenced by the philosophy of John Locke, who proposed
that the brain is like a "tabula rasa," or blank slate. According to
Locke, the brain is uniform and featureless until it receives impressions gained by experience.

The shift toward this antilocalizationist view of brain organization was strongly propelled by two American psychologists who
taught at Harvard. Karl Lashley removed different parts of rodents'
brains to see if there were areas of the brain that, when removed,
caused a specific behavioral deficit. He found no localized regions
where knowledge was stored and concluded that it seemed to be
diffusely represented. Based on these observations (later found to
be incorrect), Lashley formulated the theory of *mass action*. A cor-
ollary of this theory is that no matter where a brain injury occurs,
the more tissue that is damaged, the more poorly the animal performs. Another Harvard psychologist, B.F. Skinner, the founder of
behaviorism, thought that understanding the brain was irrelevant for
understanding behavior. He treated the brain as if it were a "black
box" and thought that the critical elements in understanding behavior were the stimulus and reinforcement (reward) patterns. Thus,
these two psychologists, among the most influential of the twentieth
century, both treated the brain as if it were a tabula rasa.

From 1920 to 1960, clinical neurologists, who presumably
should have been interested in localization of function, did little to
advance knowledge in this field. Except for a few rare individuals,
American neurologists had little interest in neuropsychology, and
many British neurologists had a strongly negative attitude toward
localizationist–connectionist thinking. Sir Henry Head, for example,
one of the leaders of British neurology during this time, wrote about
Carl Wernicke that "No better example could be chosen of the matter in which writers of this period were compelled to lop and twist
their cases to fit the Procrustean bed of their hypothetical
conceptions."

A renaissance began in 1962, when Norman Geschwind and
Edith Kaplan examined a patient with a lesion of the corpus cal-

losum. The corpus callosum carries messages between the two cerebral hemispheres. This patient was unable to carry out verbal commands with his left hand but could do so with his right hand, and he excited Geschwind's interest in neuropsychology. At the Boston Veterans Administration Hospital, Geschwind was fortunate enough to work with Fred Quadfasel, a European-trained neurologist whose mentor, Kurt Goldstein, was a student of Hugo Liepmann. Liepmann, a student of Karl Wernicke, had been the first to report a similar case of callosal disconnection in 1908. Quadfasel informed Geschwind of the important but forgotten journal articles written in French and German before the First World War. Fortunately, Geschwind was fluent in both languages. After reading these papers, he a published two-part article in *Brain* in 1965 called "Disconnexion Syndromes in Animals and Man." In this paper he synthesized the early writings, updated them on the basis of current anatomical and physiological advances, and proposed new and testable hypotheses. After the article appeared, neurologists, psychologists, speech pathologists, and other scientists began to resume the study of brain–behavior relationships, primarily by observing and testing brain-damaged patients or by presenting normal subjects with lateralized (right versus left) stimuli to study hemispheric dominance. Then the advent of new neuroimaging techniques such as computer tomography (CT) and magnetic resonance imaging (MRI) allowed clinicians and other investigators to localize lesions in living patients rather than having to rely on postmortem examination. When the nerve cells in the brain transmit information, they give off small electrical currents. Electroencephalograms (EEGs) amplify these currents, and changes in currents that are associated with specific behaviors can be recorded and used to understand which functions are being performed by different areas of the brain.

The brain requires energy. Its nerve cells get their energy by burning sugar (glucose) with oxygen, both of which are brought to the brain by blood. A particular area of the brain is activated when it is performing a specific function. With activation, blood flow to this area increases. Using various techniques, investigators can study changes in blood flow. Radioactive particles injected into the blood can be measured with positron emission tomography (PET). Because blood with and without oxygen has different magnetic properties, blood flow to an area of the brain can also be measured by inspecting these magnetic properties. Functional magnetic resonance imaging (fMRI) uses this principle to help visualize the parts of the brain that are active during different tasks. Although this technique is new, it has already taught us much about the brain and is an important source of converging evidence. In the past two decades neuropsychology and cognitive neuroscience have mushroomed, in part through the use of neuroimaging methods such as PET and fMRI, evoked potentials, and magneto-encephalography. These techniques have allowed us to perform anatomical and physiological studies of the behavior of normal people.

Clinicians now know that almost all brain diseases alter cognitive functions. This awareness and the introduction of new technology have been responsible for a phenomenal growth in neuropsychological and cognitive neuroscience research. Today there are at least five neuropsychological or cognitive neuroscience societies that have annual meetings (Academy of Aphasia, Behavioral Neurology Society, Cognitive Neuroscience Society, International Neuropsychological Society, and National Academy of Neuropsychology). The Society of Neuroscience, with over 25,000 members, also has many sessions devoted to cognitive neuroscience at its annual conventions. In addition, clinicians have become more aware of their patients' cognitive deficits, and the specialties of neurology, psychiatry, clinical psychology, and speech pathology now have subspecialists in the diagnosis and treatment of cognitive disorders. Thus, many of the traditional medical, psychological, and speech societies, such as the American Academy of Neurology, the American Psychological Association, and the American Speech and Hearing Association, also have scientific sessions where papers on neuropsychologicy are presented. Clinical journals (*Brain, Neurology, Journal of Neurology, Neurosurgery and Psychiatry, Journal of Speech and Hearing Research*, etc.) often publish neuropsychological studies. The expansion of neuropsychological research has been so great that there are now more than a dozen journals specifically devoted to such articles (*Journal of the International Neuropsychological Society, Neuropsychologia, Cortex, Behavioral Neurology, Neurocase, Journal of Cognitive Neuroscience, Cognitive Neuropsychology, Neuropsychiatry-Neuropsychology and Behavioral Neurology, Neuropsychology, Journal of Clinical Neuropsychology, Brain and Language, Brain and Cognition*). There are also many journals that, although not devoted to neuropsychology, publish numerous articles on brain–behavior relationships (*Neuroimage, Cerebral Cortex, Behav-*

ioral and Brain Sciences, Journal of Neuroscience, Science, Nature, Brain Research, Journal of Neurophysiology).

Most neuropsychological research published in journals and presented at meetings has focused on defining the behavioral and anatomical components of complex behaviors such as perception. Although there is still much to be learned about the modularity of brain and behavior, future research should also be directed at understanding the binding between modules. For example, we know that there are modules in the visual system that allow us to perceive color, form, and movement, but we do not understand how these modules are united to form a complete visual percept. Such understanding would enhance the pragmatic utility of neuropsychology. Much of the information about brain modularity has been used successfully in diagnostic tests, but the knowledge we have gained in neuropsychology and cognitive neuroscience has not had a strong influence on the rehabilitation of patients with developmental, degenerative, and lesion-induced cognitive disorders. This hybrid field is still in its infancy, and we can expect much more from it.

CHAPTER
2

LANGUAGE

Language is a complex process that allows people to communicate, reason and control behavior. Because language is unique to humans, until the recent advent of functional imaging, the primary means by which we learned about how the brain mediates language was by studying patients who had injured their brain. These studies allowed investigators to fractionate these complex processes into components and learn which portions of the brain mediate each component. Disorders of language fall into three categories: speech disorders, reading disorders, and writing disorders. We will consider each of these in turn.

SPEECH DISORDERS: APHASIA

Broca's Aphasia: Loss of Speech Programs

Although the ancients observed that diseases of the brain may interfere with language, the modern study of how the brain mediates language started with Paul Broca. In 1861, Broca, an anthropologist and physician, heard a lecture by one of Gall's students who mentioned the possibility that the memory for words was stored in the frontal lobes. (See Fig. 2–1 for a diagram of the major lobes of the brain.) At that time, Broca had a patient who was terminally ill. Before being hospitalized, the patient had lost his ability to speak. One of the few things he could say was the word *tan*. Although he could not speak spontaneously, he was able to understand speech. This patient, referred to as "Tan," died. Broca examined Tan's brain

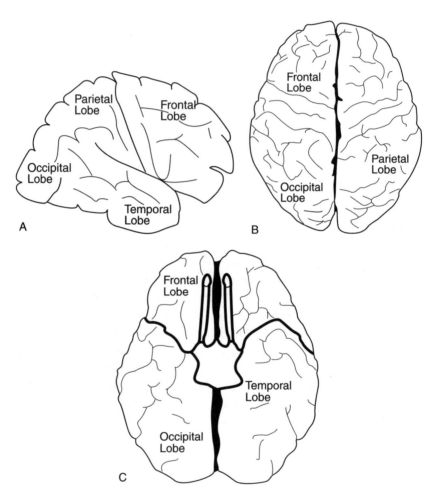

Figure 2–1. The major lobes of the brain. (A) Lateral (side) view of the brain. (B) Dorsal (top) view of the brain. (C) Ventral (bottom) view of the brain.

and found that he had had a stroke, which destroyed the left anterior portion of the brain (Fig. 2–2). Subsequently, Broca described eight patients who had lost their speech, a condition called aphasia. All of these patients were right-handed and all had weakness of their right arm, suggesting that they had suffered strokes of their left hemisphere. In his observations of these patients, Broca demonstrated not only that the anterior areas of the brain are important for programming speech sounds, but also that the left hemisphere is dominant for mediating language in right-handed people.

Automatic Speech

Shortly after arriving at the University of Florida, I saw a patient who had come from Sarasota. He and his wife had moved to Florida from Vermont a few months before he suffered a stroke that left him with Broca's aphasia and weakness of his right arm. This man had been a deacon in his church and before his stroke his wife had never heard him curse. A few weeks after his stroke, however, the only words he uttered were curses. His wife was upset about this cursing for two reasons. She thought it meant that he was angry with her, and she was afraid to have any social contact with other people because his foul language embarrassed her. She wanted to know if I could do anything for him. In addition to evaluating him to find out the cause of his stroke and help prevent future strokes, I explained

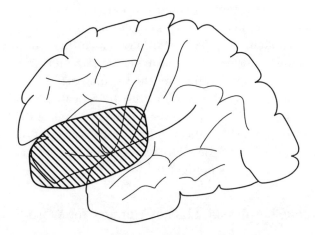

Figure 2–2. Lesion of Tan's brain, located in the inferior (lower) portion of the left frontal lobe.

to them that his inability to speak was not caused by weakness of his mouth and tongue. If weakness were causing his trouble with speaking, he would not have been able to curse. When I asked this man to sing "Jingle Bells," he sang the entire song correctly. Then I asked him to say the Lord's Prayer. I helped start him by saying, "Our Father," and he continued, "who art in heaven, hallowed be thy name. . . . " When he started saying the prayer, his wife looked amazed. When he finished the prayer, tears came to her eyes.

My mentor, Norman Geschwind, was the first to demonstrate to me that patients who could not use conversational speech could perform this type of automatic speech. This dichotomy between conversational, or propositional, speech and automatic speech was first described by a British neurologist, Hughlings Jackson, about 100 years ago. Although there has been overwhelming support for the hypothesis that the left hemisphere mediates conversational speech in right handers, the area of the brain important in automatic speech remained unknown until recently.

Several year ago, I was visiting Lynn Speedie and Eli Wertman in Israel. One of their hospital patients was a right-handed Orthodox French Jew who had recently immigrated to Israel. Several times a day Orthodox Jews chant, in Hebrew, the monotheistic prayer "Hear All Israel, the Lord Is Our God. The Lord Is One." On the day of his admission, the patient awoke and found that he could not chant this prayer, which he had recited for over 60 years; otherwise, he could converse normally. When he was tested further in the hospital, it became apparent that he could not perform other types of automatic speech and singing. For example, he loved France and had always been able to sing the French national anthem; now, however, he was unable to do so. A CT scan of the patient's brain revealed that he had had a stroke affecting the frontal part of his right hemisphere. Although this observation must be repeated by other investigators, it appears that whereas the frontal portions of the left hemisphere are important for the production of conversational speech, the frontal portions of the right hemisphere may be necessary for automatic speech and singing.

Wernicke's Aphasia: Loss of Memory for Word Sounds

In the 1960s, foreign nations could fish as close as 3 miles from the U.S. shore. A Soviet fleet was fishing nearby, and the New England fishermen were outraged; after several days of protest, the Soviets moved away. At about the same time, the police found a man wandering around Salem, Massachusetts, who, when questioned, appeared to be speaking a foreign language. They could not understand him and he, apparently unable to understand them, became progressively frustrated and angry. Because he had no identification and the police did not know what to do, they held him at the police station and called Harvard University, attempting to find a graduate student who was fluent in Russian to help them communicate with the man. The graduate student they located attempted to converse with the man but failed. The student explained to the police that many different languages were spoken in the Soviet Union and that the language spoken by the man did not sound like either a Slavic or other Indo-European language but rather one of the languages spoken near the Ural Mountains. Once again, the police called Harvard to find someone who spoke some of the Turkish languages. Another graduate student arrived and again failed to communicate with the stranger. This story was published in the local newspaper. After reading it, one of my coresidents called the Salem police to suggest that this man might have had a stroke. He explained that the stroke could have affected the posterior portion of the brain, producing no weakness or difficulty walking but leaving the man speaking what sounded like a foreign language. The police then reported that a local neurologist had already come to this man's rescue and that he did indeed have a stroke.

The first person to describe this fluent type of language disorder, or aphasia, was Carl Wernicke in 1874. Wernicke's patient had had a stroke in the posterior portion of the superior temporal gyrus (Fig 2–3). In general, sensory information travels from a specialized organ, such as the ear or eye, to a relay station deep in the brain called the *thalamus*. From the thalamus, it is transmitted to the cerebral cortex, the receiving areas of which are called *primary sensory areas*. Each sense, such as hearing or vision, has it own specialized receiving area. The primary auditory area is located in the upper part of the temporal lobe (Fig. 2–4) and performs sensory analysis. This sensory information is then sent to auditory association areas. Each sense has it own association area, and these unimodal sensory association areas are adjacent to the primary sensory area. The association areas synthesize incoming sensory information to form percepts such as the sound patterns of words.

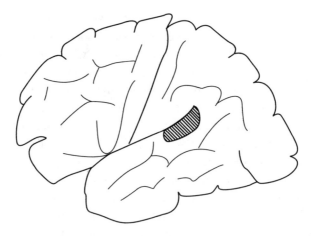

Figure 2–3. Lesion of Wernicke's area, located in the posterior (back) portion of the left superior (highest) temporal gyrus.

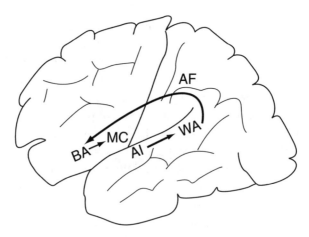

Figure 2–4. Wernicke's model of how the left hemisphere mediates speech. Auditory information enters the primary auditory cortex (A1), which is the middle part of the superior (highest) temporal lobe. After an auditory analysis, this information is relayed to the portion of the left auditory association cortex that constitutes Wernicke's area (WA). This area contains the memories of how words sound (the phonological lexicon). Wernicke's area is connected to Broca's area (BA) by a pathway called the arcuate fasiculus (AF), that is curved and travels around the back of the sylvian fissure. Broca's area is important in programming the movements necessary to produce words. It projects to the motor cortex (MC), which controls the nerves running to the muscles that move the mouth, tongue, lips, palate, and vocal chords.

The man in Salem, like the patient originally described by Wernicke, had had a stroke that destroyed the auditory association cortex on the left side. Wernicke thought that this part of the auditory association cortex contained memories, or representations, of how words sound. When this area is destroyed by a stroke, one loses the memories of how words sound and the person who loses information about how words sound not only will be unable to understand speech but also, when trying to speak, will utter nonwords, or neologisms, that are incomprehensible to the listener.

When I arrived at the University of Florida, Bob Watson showed me a patient who had Wernicke's aphasia with neologistic jargon. Although this patient used only neologisms, the prosody indicated that he was upset and wanted something. After speaking jargon for a while, he raised his voice and, out of sheer frustration, grabbed my lapels and started shaking me. Unfortunately, because these patients have lost their representations of words, they cannot even monitor their own speech and are unaware that it makes no sense. I used nonverbal gestures to calm him down.

As we discussed earlier, Gall proposed that different anatomical areas of the brain mediate different functions. Gall also thought that the size of each anatomical area was directly related to its functional capacity. Until the 1970s, most people thought that the human brain was symmetrical. Norman Geschwind, after reviewing the classic behavioral neurology literature of the nineteenth century, realized that Gall's size postulate had never been tested. Therefore, Geschwind, along with Walter Levitsky, measured the auditory association cortex behind the primary auditory area on both the right and left sides of the temporal lobes. They found that in most people this area, which includes Wernicke's area, was larger on the left side than on the right. Perhaps Gall was correct. Functions are localized, and bigger is better.

Carl Wernicke was aware of Paul Broca's seminal observations and suggested that Broca's area, located in the left frontal lobe and important in the production of speech sounds, was connected to the posterior portion of the superior temporal lobe (Wernicke's area) that stored the memories of how words sound. In order to speak, name something, or even repeat a word or sentence, one has to activate the memories of how words sound. This information can direct Broca's area to program a sequence of movements that will

The next morning during our rounds, I presented Jim Wilson to our attending neurologist, who examined the patient and asked me what I thought was wrong with him. I told him I thought he had a stroke. We moved away from the patient's bed and he asked, "How could he hear the phone ring and recognize his wife's voice but not understand words? If he was deaf he would not hear anything, and if he was aphasic he would not be able to read and speak normally."

He took me further away from the patient's bed and said, "You admitted a crock! Call psychiatry and get this faker off our service." In the 1960s, about the only words uttered by a resident to an attending physician were, "Yes, sir." I was, however, worried about this man. I told the attending physician that although I did not know much about neurology, before becoming a neurology resident I had done 4 years of internal medicine and knew that the type of artificial valve placed in this man's heart was notorious for sending emboli (blood clots) to the brain. Based on this knowledge, I had started to anticoagulate him and wanted him to be well regulated with oral medicine before we transferred him to the psychiatric service. Luckily, the attending physician agreed to let me keep him on our neurology service.

After rounds, the Chief Resident told me that Norman Geschwind, the chief of neurology at Boston University, has a strong interest in language disorders and that perhaps I should invite him to Boston City Hospital to see this patient. Traditionally on Saturday mornings we had grand rounds, and on most Saturdays we presented one or two cases to our chairman, Professor Derek Denny-Brown. This coming Saturday, however, Dr. Denny-Brown would be out of town. The Chief Resident said, "Why don't you call up Norman Geschwind and ask him if he could do rounds?" After some hesitation I called Dr. Geschwind, who agreed to my proposal.

On Saturday morning we all met in our conference room. After introducing Dr. Geschwind, I presented the patient. Dr. Geschwind examined him and found exactly what I had described. The patient could speak and name normally, but he could not understand or repeat speech. He was, however, able to understand written commands. After he completed his examination and the patient returned to his room, Dr. Geschwind explained that this man had a disorder described at the turn of the century called *pure word deafness*. He reviewed the contributions of Broca and Wernicke and then explained what would happen if the primary auditory cortex, where auditory information arrives, was injured and auditory information was unable to gain access to Wernicke's area, which contains the memories of how words sound (Fig. 2–6). Such a lesion would prevent the person from understanding spoken words, but since the visual system can gain access to the language areas, it would not prevent written language from reaching the language cortex. Because auditory signals could not enter the language cortex, repetition of speech would also be impaired, but because the remainder of the language cortex was intact, the person would be able to speak spontaneously and name normally.

Dr. Geshwind thought that Mr. Wilson's pure word deafness was caused by a stroke and that an embolus from his heart had

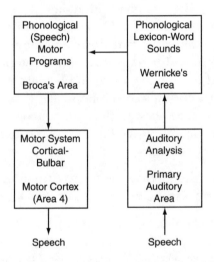

Figure 2–6. Wernicke's information-processing model. Brain injuries to the primary auditory area or its projections to Wernicke's area produce a disorder called *pure word deafness*; patients speak and name objects normally (because Wernicke's area is intact and connected to an intact Broca's area), but cannot understand speech or repeat because speech sounds cannot access Wernicke's area. When Wernicke's area is injured (Wernicke's aphasia), patients cannot comprehend, repeat, or name but have fluent speech. This speech, however, contains nonwords, or neologisms, and words that contain phonological errors, such as *gat* for *cat*. Injury to the connection between Wernicke's and Broca's areas causes conduction aphasia, in which patients can understand but, when speaking, repeating, and naming, make frequent phonological errors. Finally, injury to Broca's area induces Broca's aphasia, in which patients can understand but have trouble speaking because they cannot program their mouth, lips, tongue, palate, and vocal cords to make the correct speech sounds.

destroyed the primary auditory cortex, located just anterior to Wernicke's area. My attending physician then asked, "Norman, how was
he able to recognize that the telephone was ringing and to know
that his wife was the one who had called him?" Dr. Geschwind explained that voice and sound recognition are not verbal and
therefore can probably be mediated by the nondominant right hemisphere. In this hemisphere, the primary auditory cortex is intact and
is connected to the auditory association area and other areas of the
cortex on that side. He said that there had been reports of patients
with lesions of the primary auditory cortex on both sides. These
patients could not understand speech or recognize environmental
noises or people's voices. This disorder is called *cortical deafness.*

In 1967, there were no CT or MRI scans, but there was a new
technique for scanning the brain with radioisotopes. The technician
injected a radioisotope into the blood that circulated to the brain.
A brain scanner counted the radiation over different portions of the
brain. If the patient had had a stroke, more isotope would leak out
of the blood, and more radiation would be emitted from the areas
of the brain that were injured by the stroke than from areas that
were normal. The scan showed that the patient had had a stroke
exactly where Dr. Geschwind said it would be located.

Transcortical Sensory Aphasia: Semantic Access and Egress Deficit

In 1975 in north Florida, I saw a man who, during the hunting
season, slept in a cabin with his hunting buddy. During late autumn
it can get cold there, especially after sunset. During the night the
temperature dropped, and to keep warm the men used a kerosene
space heater. Unfortunately, the heater was not correctly vented. In
the morning some of their buddies who slept in a nearby tent came
to wake them. They found one of the two men dead and the other
comatose, with bright red skin. They immediately recognized that
the men had been poisoned by carbon monoxide. They removed
them from the cabin and called the paramedics, who gave the living
man oxygen. They then transported him to the University of Florida
Teaching Hospital for treatment in a hyperbaric chamber. Carbon
monoxide combines with red blood cells and prevents blood from
carrying oxygen to the vital organs, including the brain. Giving the
patient oxygen at high pressure forces more oxygen into the blood.

At first the patient was comatose, but after several days he regained consciousness. I was asked to see him because he had a problem with language. When I examined him, he was alert and looked directly at me. I asked him, "How are you feeling?" He replied, "How are you feeling?" I said, "Fine, thank you." He then said, "Fine, thank you." I realized that he had a condition, called *echolalia*, in which he was echoing my speech. This type of echoing is involuntary. I then attempted to test his comprehension, but he could not understand even the most simple commands, such as "Close your eyes." Occasionally he attempted to speak, but although he used English words his speech was empty. His sentences had no meaning. Some people call this condition *semantic jargon*. The patient also could not name, but he could repeat everything said to him.

Patients with the language disturbances described so far (Broca's aphasia, Wernicke's aphasia, conduction aphasia, pure word deafness) all have trouble repeating speech. Several years after Carl Wernicke described the aphasia that has been named after him, Ludwig Lichtheim described a patient whose condition was very similar to that of the patient with carbon monoxide poisoning. Lichtheim's patient appeared similar to those with Wernicke's aphasia in that he was fluent but made frequent errors. Unlike patients with Wernicke's aphasia, however, who frequently use neologisms and substitute some sounds in a word for other sounds (phonological errors), patients with this syndrome use good English words, but select the wrong words, so that their spontaneous speech carries little or no meaning. Unlike patients with Wernicke's aphasia, these patients, like the man with carbon monoxide poisoning, are able to repeat. This form of aphasia was subsequently called *transcortical sensory aphasia*. The information-processing model proposed by Wernicke cannot account for this syndrome. Lichtheim suggested that in order to understand speech, there are at least three functions that must be performed. First, one must analyze the sounds entering the brain; this function is performed by the primary auditory cortex. Next, these sounds have to activate the representation, or memories, of how words sound. As we have discussed, these memories are stored in Wernicke's area, part of the auditory association cortex, located in the posterior superior portion of the left temporal lobe. Lastly, a semantic-conceptual analysis must be performed. Lichtheim's modification of Wernicke's model is presented in Figure 2–7.

When I was in grade school, teachers often asked us what words mean. Once, when a teacher called on me, I said, "I know what that word means, but I can't explain it now." The teacher said, "If you knew what the word meant, you could give me the definition." The teacher was correct. However, in retrospect, I think I was saying that I had heard or seen this word before and knew that it was an English word that sounded or looked familiar. There are many words we read or hear that we know are good English words but we do not know their meaning. What I probably would tell my grade school teacher now is that I do have a phonological-lexical representation (recognize the sounds) of that word and I know it is a real English word, but I have not yet formed a semantic representation of it. Therefore, I do not know its meaning and cannot define it. Just as one can destroy the auditory cortex, where auditory analyses are performed, and destroy the auditory association cortex that stores memories of how words sound (lexical representations), one can either destroy semantic-conceptual representations or disconnect

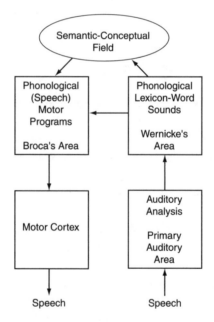

Figure 2–7. Lichtheim's modification of Wernicke's model, illustrating how the brain understands speech. After the primary auditory area performs an auditory analysis, this information activates a phonological lexical representation (memory of the speech sounds, or phonemes, that constitute learned words). In order to comprehend these lexical representations, the person must access semantic–conceptual representations.

them from the auditory association cortex. In regard to the patients who can repeat but not understand, Lichtheim suggested that in this condition semantic representations are either destroyed or disconnected from Wernicke's area (the phonological lexicon). Because these patients can perform an auditory analysis, activate memories of word sounds, and program the movements necessary to make these sounds, they can repeat. However, since they cannot perform a semantic analysis, they cannot comprehend. When they attempt to speak or name, they can activate English words, but these words are not constrained by the semantic system. Therefore, the words and sentences produced by these patients have no meaning.

In 1972 I examined Anthony Fauci, a 78-year-old man who lived with his wife in Daytona, Florida. He had suffered a stroke 2 years before I saw him. According to his wife, "he could understand things but not speech." When I tested him, he could not comprehend even the most simple sentences, but he could repeat; therefore, he appeared to have a form of transcortical sensory aphasia. Together with Ed Valenstein and Dan Tucker (the latter was then a medical student), we traveled from Gainesville to the patient's home and observed him there. He appeared to understand the world around him so long as his interactions did not depend on speech or reading. In addition to performing activities of daily living such as dressing himself and maintaining good hygiene, he was able to perform instrumental activities including using tools. Was his semantic or conceptual field destroyed or was it disconnected from the phonological lexicon? To learn if his semantic–conceptual field was destroyed, we developed a test that had a target picture and a picture that was semantically–conceptually related to the target picture. There were also two foils. One foil had a shape similar to that of the target picture; the other foil was not related to the target either semantically or visually. The task was for Mr. Fauci to point to the related picture. I showed him several examples of how to perform the task and then began the test. After each failure, I showed him the correct choice. I thought that since his semantic–conceptual field appeared to be intact, he would do extremely well on this task However, on the first five or six trials he chose the visual (similarly shaped) foil. Then we came to a trial where the target was a football, the visual foil was an eggplant, and the correct choice was goal posts. A big smile spread over his face, and he pointed to the goal posts. A big smile also spread over our faces until he did the Florida State University "chop." After this he performed correctly on almost all of the remaining trials, showing that he did understand semantic related-ness. We were so pleased with his performance that we did not draw a picture of an alligator or indicate to him that we were from the University of Florida.

Patients with severe Alzheimer's disease also may demonstrate a transcortical sensory aphasia that appears similar to that of Mr. Fauci. These patients however, often cannot perform activities of daily living or instrumental activities, and on semantic relatedness tests they perform poorly. Unlike Mr. Fauci, who had had a stroke that probably disconnected his semantic–conceptual field from his phonological lexicon, patients with Alzheimer's disease have a de-graded conceptual field.

Anomic Aphasia: Inability to Access
the Memories for Word Sounds

Lichtheim's model (Fig. 2–7) explains all the aphasic syndromes seen in the clinic except one: *anomic aphasia.* Patients with anomic aphasia have a problem naming or finding words when they are speaking. Otherwise their speech is fluent, often allowing them to describe the items whose names they cannot recall. They can repeat normally, and they can comprehend speech. Aware that his model could not explain anomic aphasia, Lichtheim denied that it ex-isted—but it does. Adolf Kussmaul, a neurologist who also worked at the turn of the twentieth century, proposed an alternative model (Fig. 2–8). Whereas Lichtheim proposed that the conceptual–se-mantic field directly activates Broca's area to produce speech, Kuss-maul stated that it directly activates the phonological lexicon (Wer-nicke's area, which contains the memories of how words sound). An impaired ability of the semantic field to gain access to the phono-logical lexicon would impair naming but leave repetition and com-prehension intact and therefore would produce the clinical picture of anomic aphasia.

Transcortical Aphasia with Intact Speech:
Inability of Word Memories to
Access Semantics

If anomic aphasia is caused by inability of the semantic–conceptual field to access the phonological lexicon, then some patients could

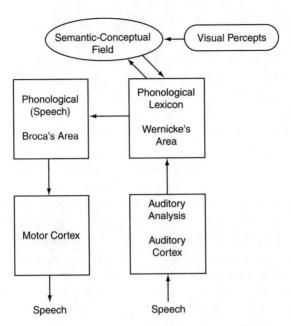

Figure 2–8. Kussmaul's model is similar to that of Lichtheim (Fig. 2–7) in that the phonological lexicon activates the semantic–conceptual field so that people can comprehend speech. However, when a person wants to speak spontaneously, name an object (after recognizing an object), or express a thought, according to Kussmaul, the semantic–conceptual field activates the phonological lexicon, which contains the memories of the word sounds that represent the object to be named or the thought to be expressed. In Kussmaul's model, as in Lichtheim's, injury to the areas of the brain that perform auditory analysis (primary auditory cortex), the phonological lexicon (Wernicke's area), or the semantic–conceptual field interferes with comprehension. However, if an intact semantic–conceptual field cannot access the phonological lexicon, the patient will be unable to name objects or speak normally, but the person can comprehend (because auditory information can access the semantic–conceptual field). The patient can also repeat because the auditory information can access the phonological lexicon (Wernicke's area), the phonological lexicon can access Broca's area, which programs the movements needed to make speech sounds, and Broca's area can excite the motor cortex, which controls the muscles of the mouth. If, in contrast, the semantic–conceptual field can access the phonological lexicon (Wernicke's area) but Wernicke's area cannot access the semantic–conceptual field, the patient will be able to name and speak but not comprehend speech.

have the oppposite condition. In this disorder, the phonological lexicon could have difficulty accessing the semantic–conceptual field,
but the semantic field could access the phonological lexicon and
Broca's area. While I was the attending physician in our inpatient
service, the neurology resident presented the following patient: "Mr
Lamar Jones is a 67-year-old man who has been relatively healthy his
entire life, except that he has mild hypertension that has been
treated with hydrochlorothiazide. Last night he was home with his
wife watching television. Suddenly, he and his wife noticed that he
had trouble speaking and understanding his wife's speech. Because
he did not improve in 4 hours, his wife drove him to the emergency
room. I examined him. His vital signs were good, including his
blood pressure, which was 140/80. His heart sounded normal. His
heart rhythm was normal, and he did not have murmurs. However,
he did have a high-pitched bruit [the sound made by fluid being
pushed through a narrow opening] over his left carotid artery. The
remainder of his general physical examination was normal. His entire neurological examination was also normal except for mental
status testing. The patient had great difficulty understanding commands. He also had difficulty speaking and naming objects. When
he spoke his speech was fluent, but he made a lot of errors in which
he used the wrong words, so he was very difficult to understand.
However, his repetition was perfect." I asked the resident, "What did
you have him repeat?" He replied, "No ifs, ands, or buts." I then
asked, "What do you think happened to this man?" He said, "I am
not sure, but I think that his language problem seems to be a transcortical sensory aphasia from a watershed infarction [stroke]
caused by a thrombosis of the left internal carotid artery [one of
the major vessels that carries blood to the brain]." A CT scan showed
nothing abnormal. I reminded him that sometimes it takes several
day before anything appears on a CT scan. We then went to the
patient's bedside so that I could examine him. My findings on the
physical and general neurological examinations agreed with those
of the resident. However, when I asked the patient how he was feeling, he replied, "Doctor, this young doctor took real good care of
me. I also appreciate you taking care of me, but I want to go home.
I do not like hospitals and do not like the food in this place." Almost all aphasic patients have abnormal speech, so I said to the resident, "This man's spontaneous speech is normal. I guess he is no
longer aphasic. I wonder if this was a transient ischemic attack, with

no permanent damage?" I then told the patient, "We have thinned your blood, and tomorrow I would like you to have an angiogram. This angiogram will tell us if we need to operate on a blood vessel that goes to your brain. If this blood vessel is too narrow, the surgeon may be able to repair it. Do you have any question that you would like to ask me?" He looked up at me and said, "Doctor I like to go fishing . . . for bass." Because of this reply, I became suspicious that he might not be understanding me and decided to test his comprehension. I put five common objects (pen, dollar, wallet, watch, and credit card) on a table in front of him and said, "Please point to the pen." He looked at me with a puzzled expression and said, "I can hear you talking, but I can't understand what you are saying." I continued to test his comprehension by asking him to point to various objects. After I showed him how to point he did so, but his pointing was totally random, so only about 20% of the attempts were correct. It was remarkable how well he spoke but how poorly he comprehended. Equally remarkable was his naming. I held up one object at a time, and he appeared to understand that I wanted the objects named. In spite of being unable to understand the names of these objects, he named all of them correctly. His repetition, as the resident suggested, was totally intact. It appeared that he had a transcortical sensory aphasia with intact spontaneous speech and naming. I had never seen this combination of symptoms and knew of no reports of it. When the resident apologized for saying that the patient's speech and naming were abnormal, I said that patients often change after they are admitted to the hospital. The next day the patient did have an angiogram, which demonstrated that his carotid artery on the left side was totally occluded. Unfortunately, no surgical repair was possible. We did provide him with speech therapy and medicines that we hoped would prevent further strokes.

The observations we made on this most unusual patient were important because they further supported the Kussmaul model (Fig. 2–8). They also demonstrated that the phonological lexicon may have trouble accessing the semantic–conceptual field, thereby impairing comprehension, but that the semantic–conceptual field could access the phonological lexicon, permitting the patient to name and to speak spontaneously.

Transcortical Motor Aphasia: Inability
to Activate Semantics

Although Kussmaul's model accounted for all the types of aphasia
we have discussed, there are two observations that it cannot explain.
Lichtheim described a patient who had difficulty initiating speech
and was therefore nonfluent. This patient's nonfluency was similar
to that of someone with Broca's aphasia. In addition, like Broca's
aphasics, this patient could comprehend speech. However, unlike
Broca's aphasics, repetition was excellent and the patient could
name extremely well. This disorder is called transcortical motor
aphasia. According to Lichtheim's model (Fig. 2–7), it is caused by
a disconnection between the semantic–conceptual field and Broca's
area. Using Lichtheim's model, one would expect that after formu-
lating a concept, the inability to activate the programs needed to
create phonemes would cause nonfluency. However, since patients
with this disconnection can perform an auditory–phonological–lexical analysis and activate the conceptual–semantic network, they
should be able to comprehend. Because they can perform an auditory–phonological–lexical analysis and the lexicon can access Broca's
area and the motor cortex, the patient should be able to repeat.
However, one of the problems with Lichtheim's model is that it cannot explain why some of these patients can name well. We therefore
considered modifying Kussmaul's model. As I will discuss in Chapter
9, the frontal lobes are very important in the initiation of behavior.
Patients with frontal lobe lesions often fail to initiate actions, a condition called *akinesia* (without movement). The lesions associated
with transcortical motor aphasia are usually located in the left frontal lobe superior to Broca's area or in the medial surface of the
frontal lobes (Fig. 2–9). Injury to these frontal lobe regions may
induce a deficit of intention in which patients cannot activate their
conceptual–semantic field spontaneously. They need an external
stimulus to activate this field. Our modification of Kussmaul's model
is presented in Figure 2–10.

Optic Aphasia: Inability of Visual Percepts
to Access Word Sound Memories

Mrs. Block, a 72-year-old retired school teacher, had been working
in an art museum as a tour guide. One day she noticed that she was

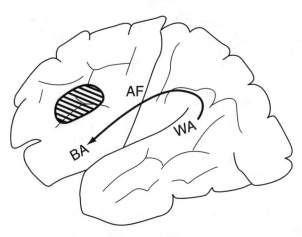

Figure 2–9. Diagram of the area in the frontal lobe that may be injured when patients have transcortical motor aphasia with a reduced ability to speak spontaneously (nonfluent speech) and with intact comprehension and repetition (WA = Wernicke's area; BA = Broca's area; AF = arcuate fasiculus).

having difficulty finding the names of artists whose paintings were hanging in the museum, as well as the people and objects depicted in these paintings. Her general physical and neurological examinations were normal, except that she had trouble seeing things in the right upper quarter of her visual field. This problem, which affected both eyes, is often caused by damage to the lower portion of the visual cortex on the left side. When I tested her naming ability by holding up objects and asking her to name them, she had trouble doing so. She appeared to know, however, what these objects were because she could describe their use. For example, she had trouble naming common objects like a pen and a watch but said, "That's the thing you write with and that is a thing for keeping time." Her inability to name objects appeared to be similar to the defects we see with anomic aphasia, but unlike the patient with anomic aphasia, she did not have trouble finding names while speaking spontaneously. In addition, when I asked her to close her eyes and put the same objects in her hand that she could not name by sight, she named all the objects correctly. Patients with anomic aphasia have trouble naming objects in all modalities. The disorder this patient was demonstrating is called *optic aphasia.* The Kussmaul model (Fig. 2–8) cannot account for this disorder. According to the model, one names visually presented objects by having the visual percept activate

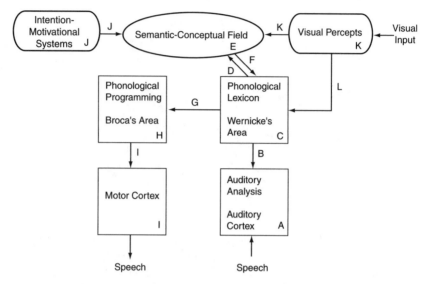

Figure 2–10. Our modification of Kussmaul's model. In this model the frontal lobe, which is responsible for initiating behaviors, may be important in activating the semantic–conceptual field. When the left frontal lobe is injured semantic activation fails, producing transcortical motor aphasia, in which the patient cannot initiate speech but can repeat. This model also attempts to illustrate all the possible speech language functions. In order to comprehend speech, one would use the system represented by A, B, C, D, E. To repeat, one would use the system represented by A, B, C, G, H, I. To speak spontaneously, one would use the system represented by J, E, F, C, G, H, I. To name, one would use the system represented by K, E, F, C, G, H, I. Interruption of these systems would also impair the functions that they mediate. Therefore, this model also accounts for all of the aphasic (speech and language) disorders induced by brain injury.

the semantic–conceptual field; this field then accesses the phonological lexicon, where the memories of word sounds are stored. Using this model, the only possible explanation is that vision could not access semantics but other sensory modalities, such as touch, could. However, Mrs. Block could not find the names for visually presented objects but she did know their use, demonstrating that visual information can access semantics. A modification of Kussmaul's model may allow us to explain this visual modality–specific naming defect. Perhaps, as illustrated in Figure 2–10, visual percepts access not only the semantic–conceptual field but also the phonological lexicon (Wernicke's area), and Wernicke's area activates Broca's area to produce the names of the objects. In patients who have optic aphasia, the visual percept cannot access the phonological lexicon directly, but it can access the semantic–conceptual field.

If I presented two different nonsense shapes, stated that one was a *framazoid* and the other was a *flig*, and then asked subjects to point to the flig, I believe that almost all normal people would be able to learn these visual percept–phonological associations. Because these are nonsense shapes, there are no semantic representations. Our ability to name these shapes suggests that we are able to perform cross-modal (visual to auditory) associations and demonstrates that visual percepts may be able to access the phonological lexicon directly.

Non-optic Aphasia: Inability of Visual Percepts to Access Semantics

Kussmaul's model, and our modification of it, could not explain the disorder in a patient we saw in our Memory Disorder Clinic. He was a 67-year-old retired electrical engineer who had a 3-year history of memory and language problems that, according to his wife, was slowly progressive. When we tried to get a history from this man, he used semantic jargon consisting of standard English words, but the sentences were empty of meaning. His comprehension of verbal commands was also severely impaired, and he could not even understand the most simple commands, such as "Point to the ceiling." His repetition, however, was flawless. In order to test his naming, we used the Boston Naming Test. In this test the patient is shown 60 pictures of objects like a bed, a volcano, and an abacus. After seeing the pictures, the patient is instructed to state the names of the objects. Normal people who take this test usually are able to name more than 50 items, but people with impaired naming get fewer than 50. To our surprise, this man was able to name 59 of the 60 objects. According to Kussmaul's model (Fig. 2–8), after one sees an object and this visual information accesses the conceptual–semantic field for meaning, this field accesses the phonological lexicon for memories of how words sound and then Broca's area for speech programming. This patient could not comprehend speech and could not correctly speak spontaneously, suggesting either that his conceptual–semantic field was degraded or that his phonological lexicon had been disconnected from his semantic–conceptual field, preventing the field from gaining access to his store of word sounds. In either case, according to Kussmaul's model, a person with a degraded semantic–conceptual field or a disconnected lexicon should not be able to name almost flawlessly. That this man, and two other similar patients, could name almost perfectly provides further evidence that visual percepts may have direct access to the phonological lexicon without first activating conceptual–semantic representations.

Summary

Right-handed people use their left hemisphere to speak and understand. By contrast, the majority of left-handed people are left hemisphere–dominant, but some are right hemisphere–dominant and others use both hemispheres to speak and understand. Within the left hemisphere, the lower posterior portion of the left frontal lobe is important in programming speech sounds (Broca's area). When the individual listens to speech, after the primary auditory area performs an auditory analysis, this information activates the phonological lexicon (Wernicke's area), located in the posterior portion of the superior temporal lobe. Wernicke's area contains the memories of the speech sounds that make up words. For the individual to comprehend speech, these phonological lexical representations must also access semantic–conceptual representations.

If a person wants to speak spontaneously or name an object, the semantic–conceptual field, which contains the thoughts the person wants to communicate, activates the phonological lexicon, which then accesses Broca's area. The diagrammatic model that summarizes the distributed modular speech system and the aphasic disorders induced by disruption of this system can be found in Figure 2–10.

Selected Reading

Benson, D.F., (1993) Aphasia. In *Clinical neuropsychology*. (Ed.) Heilman, K.M., and Valenstein, E., Oxford University Press, New York, pp. 17–36.

Caplan, D.N. (1987) *Neurolinguistics and linguistic aphasia*, Cambridge University Press, New York.

Geschwind, N. (1965) Disconnexion syndromes in animals and man. *Brain* 88:237–294, 585–644.

Goodglass, H. (1993) *Understanding aphasia,* Academic Press, New York.

Goodglass, H., Kaplan, E. (1972) *The assessment of aphasia and related disturbances,* Lea & Febiger, Philadelphia.

Hecean, H., Albert, M.L. (1978) *Human neuropsychology,* Wiley, New York.

Nadeau, S.E., Rothi, L.J.G., Crosson, B. (2000) *Aphasia and language,* Guilford Press, New York.

READING DISORDERS: ALEXIA OR DYSLEXIA

There are patients who have impaired speech comprehension but are able to read normally and vice versa, suggesting that the portions of the brain that mediate speech and reading comprehension are independent. In this section I discuss how the brain recognizes and understands written language by describing patients who lost this ability.

Pure Alexia: Inability to See Words

Tom Feldman, the 61-year-old president of a small environmental engineering firm in Gainesville, was diabetic and had hypertension. At the age of 55 he had suffered a heart attack but had been doing well until the day we saw him in the hospital. He awoke, as usual, at 5:30 A.M., worked out on his Nordic Track, and then took a shower, shaved, dressed and went to work, arriving there by 7:30 A.M. because he wanted to perform some dictation before the secretaries came in. He had no trouble dictating. About 8:15 one of the secretaries phoned and asked if she could bring an important letter for him to sign. He told her to come right in. She handed him the letter to sign, but when he tried to read it he could see some of the printed letters but could not read the words. He asked his secretary if the typing looked normal to her, and she said yes, it looked fine. Although he could not read the typed words, he was embarrassed to tell the secretary, so he signed the letter without having read it, something he had never done.

As soon as his secretary left, Mr. Feldman called his doctor to report this strange symptom, but the doctor was still making rounds and was unavailable. The nurse who answered the phone gave Mr. Feldman three options. He could wait until the doctor returned and called him back, he could call his ophthalmologist, or he could go to the emergency room. The ophthalmologist was in the operating room that morning so Tom went to the emergency room. The nurse there checked his vital signs and blood sugar level. Both were within the normal range. An emergency room physician listened to his heart and lungs and then called for a neurology consultation. One of our residents saw him and decided to admit him because he thought that Mr. Feldman had suffered a stroke.

When I examined him about an hour later, he demonstrated several abnormalities. He could not see my fingers when he was looking straight ahead and my hand was on his right side. This half-sided blindness, called *hemianopia*, was present in both eyes. For example, when I told him to look at my nose and tell me if I was wiggling the fingers of my left hand, my right hand, or was not wiggling any fingers, he had no trouble seeing the fingers of my right hand that were on his left side, but he could not see the wiggling fingers of my left hand that were on his right side. He also had memory problems. Although he knew where he was and could name the date, he could only recall one of three objects that I told him to remember (daisy, lamp, and mirror) after he was distracted by counting backward from 100 by sevens. When I tested his reading, it was immediately apparent that he had trouble reading. The first word I wrote on a piece of paper was *dog.* He looked at this word for a few seconds and then uttered the names of each of the letters out loud: "*D* [dee], *O* [oh], *G* [gee]." Then he repeated these three letters several times and finally said the word *dog.* When I gave him other short words, he did the same thing, first saying the letters out loud and finally saying the word. Although he could use this spelling-out-loud strategy for short words, when I asked him to read longer words or entire sentences, he had difficulty reading the words. Tests of other visual functions showed that he could recognize objects like a watch, a pen, and a wallet. I showed him some pictures of famous people cut out of a magazine, and he had no trouble recognizing them, making some disparaging remarks about politicians who were Democrats. Then I showed him large sheets of colored paper and asked him to name their color. He could not name the correct color.

For example, he called the red sheet blue and the blue sheet yellow. Next, I gave him about 20 small pieces of colored paper. There were ten colors, with two pieces of paper for each color. I mixed the order of the pieces of paper, spread them out on a table in front of him, and asked him to put the same colored pieces of paper together. While he could not name the colors, he could easily match all ten pieces of paper with their color mate. This test demonstrated that his inability to name colors was not caused by a visual disorder.

Although Mr. Feldman was unable to read normally, he speech was normal and he could write quite well. After he wrote several sentences on different pieces of paper, I selected one piece of paper, showed it to him, and asked him to read what he had written. He was able to recognize his handwriting, but he was unable to read what he had written.

The first person to describe this clinical picture, at the beginning of the twentieth century, was the French neurologist Joseph Jules Dejerine. Dejerine's patient had had a stroke of the left occipital lobe (see Fig.2–11), and when we performed MRI scans of Mr. Feldman's brain, we found that he had a lesion in the same area of the occipital lobe.

Dejerine was aware of the work of Broca, who had demonstrated that it is the left hemisphere that mediates language. The language areas described by Broca and Wernicke are next to the sylvian fissure, which separates the temporal lobe from both the parietal and frontal lobes (Fig.2–1) but Mr. Feldman's lesion was located in the occipital lobe, which was remote from these language areas. Dejerine suggested that with a lesion of the left occipital lobe (which is the area of the cortex that receives visual information from the left side of the retina of both eyes), the patient would be unable to see the words that fell on his or her right side. However, that person would be able to see the words that fell on the right side of the retina from the left visual field, because the words would reach the intact right occipital cortex. Normally, items seen by the right occipital cortex can be transferred to the left hemisphere by the major cable that connects the two hemisphere, called the *corpus callosum* (Fig. 2–11). Unfortunately, the injury to the left occipital lobe also prevents the visual information from the right hemisphere from reaching the left hemisphere's language areas. According to Dejerine, a left occipital lesion disconnects vision from the language areas, and this disconnection causes pure alexia. This same mechanism

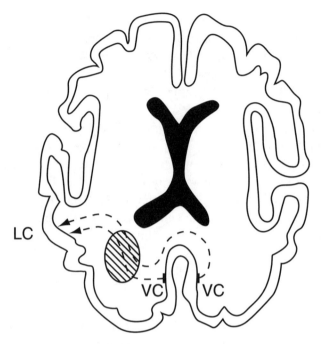

Figure 2–11. Diagram of a lesion that causes pure alexia (an inability to read with a preserved ability to write). The arrows demonstrate the flow of information from the left and right visual cortices (VC) in the occipital lobes to the language cortex (LC) in the left hemisphere. The lesion in the left occipital lobe prohibits the visual information from gaining access to the language areas.

may account for Mr. Feldman's inability to name colors. Although the colors can be seen by the right occipital cortex, the lesion of the left occipital lobe prevents transfer of this information to the language areas in the left hemisphere where the names of the colors are stored. Mr. Feldman could match colors because matching does not require language.

When a person has to name an object or a face, one would expect this visual information to follow the same route as written words, from visual cortex to language areas, but Mr. Feldman and other patients like him with pure alexia can name objects and famous faces better than they can read or name colors. The reason for this dissociation is not known, but some behavioral neurologists think that the information about objects and faces may travel more forward in the right hemisphere before it crosses the corpus callosum. Thus, an occipital lesion that impairs the function of the visual cortex and prevents the information from crossing the most posterior part of the corpus callosum (the splenium) may not prevent other information that passes across more anteriorly from reaching the left hemisphere.

When patients like Mr. Feldman are asked to pronounce words spelled to them by the examiner, they can name the words. They can perform this task correctly because they still have the memory of the letters that make up words. Although they cannot access this information visually, they can access it auditorally. Each letter in the English alphabet has a name and is a symbol for a sound. Patients like Mr. Feldman may name letters aloud because they are treating the letters as objects and are naming these objects in order to spell to themselves, bypassing their visual–language disconnection.

Phonological Dyslexia: Inability to Convert Written Letters to Speech Sounds

There are two strategies we can use to read words. Each letter has a specific sound associated with that letter. Some speech sounds, like *th* in words like *that*, require two letters, and some letters have more than one sound, like the *a* in *at* versus the *a* in *ate*. The letter or letters that are symbols for sounds are called *graphemes*, and the speech sounds that make up words are called *phonemes*. To learn how a printed word sounds, a person may translate or transcode each grapheme into its phoneme. This grapheme-to-phoneme transcoding method of reading is used mainly when we first learn to read and when we see words that we do not recognize. For example, if I ask you to pronounce the nonword *frinomin*, you may find that you are using this grapheme-to-phoneme system. However, when a person attempts to read irregular words like *yacht* by using this system, the person will read the word incorrectly. To read irregular words, one must use a whole-word or lexical system. Most normal readers use both the grapheme-to-phoneme transcoding system and the whole-word system. However, in the clinic, we have seen patients with strokes affecting the left hemisphere who could not read using the grapheme-to-phoneme system but could use the whole-word method and others who could not use the whole-word method but could use the grapheme-to-phoneme system. Patients with the former problem (who are unable to convert graphemes to phonemes) have the disorder called *phonological dyslexia*. Because most people who are experienced readers can use the whole-word method, loss of the ability to convert graphemes to phonemes usually does not cause a severe disability. However, when they have to learn new words or when they read a word they have heard before but have not seen, they have to use the grapheme-to-phoneme system. Although phonological dyslexia in adults may cause only minor reading problems, if a child who is learning to read cannot convert graphemes to phonemes, he or she may never be able to develop a memory store of whole-word sounds (orthographic lexicon) and therefore may never develop reading skills. The most common cause of developmental dyslexia is the inability to convert letters to their speech sounds or phonological dyslexia.

Lexical Dyslexia: Inability to Read Whole Words

Because the whole-word system can be used to read both irregular and regular words, patients who have lost the ability to read whole words may be severely reading impaired. We have found that in many of these patients, the left angular gyrus has been destroyed (Fig. 2–12). Just as Wernicke's area, located in the posterior portion of the superior temporal gyrus, contains the memories of how learned words sound (the phonological lexicon), the angular gyrus is believed to contain the memories of how words look (the reading or orthographic lexicon).

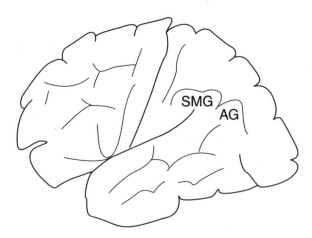

Figure 2–12. Diagram of the left hemisphere's angular gyri (AG) and supramarginal (SMG) gyri.

Several years ago, we saw Mr. Jackson, a 72-year-old man with Wernicke's aphasia from a stroke confined to the left posterior portion of the superior temporal lobe (Wernicke's area). Like the patients we described in the "Speech" section, he was unable to comprehend speech. When he was in the hospital immediately after his stroke, he was also unable to understand written language. About 2 weeks after he went home, his wife was preparing chicken for dinner. Since his stroke, his wife was trying to keep him on a low-cholesterol diet. Because he did not like fish, she cooked chicken for him almost every evening. As she was preparing the chicken, she saw him looking for a book on the shelves. She observed him as he appeared to thumb through the pages. Then he put his index finger on a particular page and brought it to his wife. His finger pointed to the word *steak*. His wife, who was unable to communicate with him, wrote a message: "Would you like me to go to the store and get you a steak?" He nodded. Although she knew she was breaking his diet, she was so happy that she had found a means to communicate with him that she returned the chicken to the refrigerator and drove him to the store to let him select a steak. After he finished the steak and fries, he open his dictionary to the *D* section and pointed to the word *delicious*.

Mr. Jackson was able to recognized written words but not spoken words because the memories, or representations, of spoken words (phonological lexicon) were destroyed by his stroke but his memories, or representations, of written words (orthographic lexicon) were preserved. Normally, after a word is recognized by the area of the brain that stores written word images (the orthographic lexicon), the activated representation can access either the semantic networks for word meaning or the phonological lexicon for pronunciation or reading aloud. Because Mr. Jackson's phonological lexicon was destroyed, he could not read aloud but could comprehend.

Semantic Dyslexia: Reading Aloud Without Understanding

There are patients with intact orthographic and phonological representations who can read aloud but not understand, because either their semantic fields are degraded or their phonological and orthographic representations are disconnected from semantics and therefore cannot access semantics. For example, I often write simple

commands for these patients to follow, such as "Point to the ceiling."
These patients will read the command but fail to carry out the action. I will then write, "Please do what this command requests. Point
to the ceiling." Again these patients will read the command out loud
but will not carry it out. Because their phonological lexicon cannot

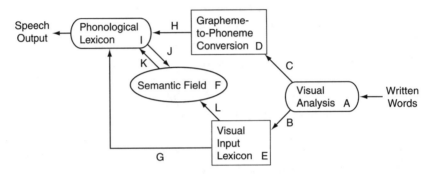

Figure 2–13. Diagrammatic model of the reading process. The images of
words and letters are projected to the occipital lobe where they undergo visual
analysis (A). This analysis allows the person to recognize the forms of the letters
and their groupings to form words. After visual analysis, the words can be processed by two different routes. In the grapheme-to-phoneme route, each word
is broken into its component letters, or graphemes. The reader then finds the
speech sound, or phoneme, represented by each grapheme (D). The reader
puts these sounds together to form a word, and this word activates the word
sound representation in the phonological lexicon (I). The phonological lexicon
(Wernicke's area) contains the memories, or representations, of how words
sound. The phonological lexicon allows the person to speak the word or learn
its meaning by accessing the semantic–conceptual field (F). An alternative
means of reading is the whole-word reading system. Representations of the visual images of words are stored in the visual input lexicon (E). After visual
analysis, these whole-word visual memories are activated. They then access the
semantic–conceptual field (F) for meaning or the phonological lexicon (I) for
speech. Disorders of the grapheme-to-phoneme system (C, D, H, I) prevent
patients from reading aloud either new words or pseudowords (e.g., *flig*), a
disorder called *phonological dyslexia*. Disorders of the whole-word system (BE)
prevent patients from reading irregular words (e.g., *yacht*). Injury to both systems prevents them from reading all types of words. Injury to the semantic–
conceptual field (F) or an inability to access this field (L, K) allows the patient
to read aloud but not comprehend what he or she has read. Patients in whom
the visual input lexicon (E) is dissociated from the phonological lexicon (I)
can understand written irregular words (e.g., *yacht*) but, when reading aloud,
they may make semantic errors (e.g., read aloud *boat* instead of *yacht*). This
disorder is called *deep dyslexia*.

access the semantic net, these patients can also repeat a spoken command, but they cannot understand spoken language and therefore do not follow the command. A diagrammatic model of these processes and how they may break down is presented in Figure 2–13.

Summary

Two strategies can be used to read words. Each letter or group of letters has a specific sound associated with it. The letter or letters that are symbols for sounds are called *graphemes,* and the speech sounds that make up words are called *phonemes.* To learn how a printed word sounds, a person may translate each grapheme into its phoneme. This grapheme-to-phoneme transcoding method of reading is used mainly when we first learn to read and when we see words that we do not recognize. A person who attempts to read irregular words by using the grapheme-to-phoneme system would read the word incorrectly. Thus, to read irregular words, one must use the whole-word system. Most normal readers use both the grapheme-to-phoneme system and the whole-word system. Reading, like speech, is mediated by the left hemisphere. The reading systems are parallel and independent but interactive with the speech systems. Just as Wernicke's area, located in the posterior portion of the superior temporal gyrus, contains the memories of how learned words sound, the angular gyrus contains the memories of how words look (the reading, or orthographic, lexicon). A diagrammatic model of the reading system is presented in Figure 2–13.

Selected Readings

Coltheart, M., Patterson, K.E., Marshall, J. (Eds.), (1980) *Deep dyslexia,* Routledge and Kegan Paul, London.

Coslett, H.B. (1997) Acquired alexia. In *Behavioral neurology and neuropsychology.* (Ed.) Feinberg, T.E., and Farah, M.J., McGraw-Hill, New York, pp. 197–208.

Friedman, R.P., Ween, J.E., Albert, M.L. (1993) Alexia. In *Clinical neuropsychology.* (Ed.) Heilman, K.M., and Valenstein, E. Oxford University Press, New York, pp. 37–62.

Geschwind, N. (1965) Disconnexion syndromes in animals and man. *Brain* 88:237–294, 585–644.

McCarthy, R.A., Warrington, E.K. (1990) Reading. In *Cognitive neuropsychology.* Academic Press, New York, pp. 214–240.

Writing Disorders: Agraphia or Dysgraphia

Disorders of writing can be dissociated from both speech (aphasia) and reading (alexia) disorders. Thus, while the speech, reading, and writing systems are interactive, they also are independent. In this section, I discuss the brain mechanisms that mediate writing.

Callosal Agraphia: An Interhemispheric Disconnection Disorder

After graduating from high school, John Thomas enlisted in the Army during the Korean War. He took his basic training at Fort Dix, New Jersey, and was sent to Korea. He fought on the front lines for several months. After the war ended, he was stationed at Fort Benning, Georgia. One day he received an announcement that enlisted servicemen who were interested in attending college should go to Building C to be tested. He took a test that lasted for several hours. He did not think he did very well, but about a month later he was informed that he had gotten one of the highest grades. He had grown up in Alabama and always wanted to go to Auburn University. The Army sent him to Auburn, and he became a civil engineer. After receiving his B.S. degree, he returned to the Army and had a 30-year career with the Army Corps of Engineers, including serving twice in Vietnam. He was the first member of his family to get a college education, and he was extremely proud when he was promoted to the rank of full colonel. On reaching the age of 65, he retired. He wanted to return to Alabama or even live in Colombus, Georgia, but his wife's family lived in the Jacksonville, Florida area, so they bought a home on the beach and retired. Before retirement he was, according to his wife, a social drinker, which usually meant two bourbons and water before dinner. After retirement, however, his alcohol consumption increased and within 6 months he had started to drink bourbon and water immediately after breakfast and continued drinking until he fell asleep on the couch at night. At first he volunteered at the Boys Club and tried to learn golf, but each week his wife noticed that he spent more and more time in front of the television set, something he had rarely done before except to watch the evening news. Finally, before his wife brought him to Gainesville Veteran's Hospital, he sat on the couch and did not even turn on the television set. He even kept a bottle of bourbon and a pitcher of water next to him so that he did not have to leave the couch to refill his glass.

In the emergency room, his wife told the physician the story of his Army career, his retirement, his drinking, and his lack of interest in doing anything except drinking. She told the doctor that she thought he was extremely depressed. The physician gave Colonel Thomas an injection of 100 mg thiamine because sometimes people who drink excessive amounts of alcohol do not absorb this vitamin, which can damage the brain. The doctor performed a brief general examination, which was normal, and ordered some laboratory tests, such as a thyroid function test to make certain that there was no physical or metabolic reason for this man's inactivity. When the emergency room physician found that all these tests were normal he called a psychiatrist, who came to see the colonel and admitted him with the diagnosis of depression. In addition to receiving daily psychotherapy, he was started on an antidepressant. After taking the drug for several weeks, he showed no improvement. The dose was then increased, but with no result. Other antidepressants were tried, but after about 6 weeks in the hospital, there was not the slightest improvement. As a last resort, the physicians decided to try treating him with electroshock therapy (ECT). This treatment often works in people who are resistant to the other forms of therapy that the colonel had undergone.

Before treating the colonel with ECT, his psychiatrist wanted to make certain that he had no neurological disease that could be causing his inertia, also called *abulia*. The psychiatrist ordered an MRI scan of his brain. The radiologist found only mild brain atrophy consistent with a man of his age. Even though the MRI scan was reported as normal, the psychiatrist wanted to make certain that there was no brain damage and requested a neurology consultation. When we examined the colonel, we noticed that he performed very poorly on tests of frontal lobe function. For example, when asked to name, in 1 minute, as many words as possible that start with the letter *A*, but no proper names, he was able to give only three words (*army, artillery, airplane*). Normal people should be able to name at least 12 words that start with the letter *A*. In addition, when we tried to engage him in a conversation, he usually gave only one-word responses. He also had abnormal reflexes, suggesting that his frontal lobes were not working properly. For example, we asked him not to grasp or hold our hands, but every time we rubbed our fingers against his palm, he grabbed our fingers and held them. This action is called the *grasp reflex*. A similar reflex can be observed in infants, but as they mature, it normally disappears. However, if the frontal lobes are not working properly, this reflex may return.

Italian neurologists have described a disorder, associated with drinking Italian red wine, that is very similar to the one the colonel was demonstrating. This disorder is called *Marchiafava-Bignami disease*. This rare disorder has now been described in almost all racial and ethnic groups that have abused many different types of alcoholic beverages. In addition to having frontal lobe dysfunction, patients with this disorder develop a cyst in the corpus callosum (Fig. 2–14). Because these cysts are associated with dysfunction of the corpus callosum, I decided to test the colonel's callosal function by asking him to write with both his right and left hands. He asked us what topic to write about, and I suggested the weather. With his right-hand he wrote, "Sunny." I then asked him to write what he did for a living with his left hand. He said, "I am right-handed." We asked

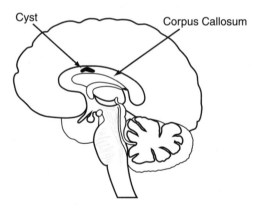

Figure 2–14. Diagram of a cyst in the corpus callosum. The corpus callosum connects the right and left hemispheres. The representations of the motor programs needed to write letters are stored in the left hemisphere. The cyst in the corpus callosum prevents these motor representations from gaining access to the motor areas of the right hemisphere. As a result, the person with this callosal lesion cannot write correctly with the left hand.

him to try. He had difficulty holding the pencil with his left hand. He was trying to write the word *Army* but the letters were formed almost by trial and error. All the letters were extremely distorted; however, they were correct. After he wrote "Army" with his left hand he said, "See, I am right-handed."

Although people with a right-hand preference do write better with their right than with their left hand, normal right handers can form legible letters with their left hand; however, the colonel's letters were not very legible. Based on my examination, I told his psychiatrist that I thought he had Marchiafava-Bignami syndrome. The psychiatrist asked, "How could that be? His MRI was read as normal." The resident and I went to the radiology department to see the films. The radiologist who had read them was there and put them on the view box for us. They revealed a large cyst in the anterior part of the corpus callosum indicative of Marchiafava-Bignami syndrome.

The type of abulia that Colonel Thomas was demonstrating is often associated with damage to the medial part of the frontal lobes, and the MRI scan showed that this area was also abnormal. However, it was probably the cystic degeneration of the anterior or front portion of the corpus callosum the was causing the colonel's problem in writing with his left hand. Writing requires at least two skills. When learning to print or write, a person has to learn the movements that are used to form letters. Most of us learned this skill so long ago that we may not recall how difficult it is. In most right handers, like the colonel, the memories, or representations, of how to make these skilled movements are stored in the left hemisphere. The second thing we must learn in order to write is how to spell words. This information, as we will discuss shortly, is also stored in the left hemisphere. The corpus callosum is the main "cable" by which information from the left hemisphere reaches the right hemisphere. Because the colonel normally could write with his right hand, his memories of how to spell words and how to form letters were both intact and could reach the motor area of the left hemisphere that controls the right hand. However, because alcohol abuse had caused damage to his corpus callosum, the information on how to form letters could not be transmitted from his left to his right hemisphere. However, the right side of his brain did know the letters that were needed to spell *Army*, so that information was able to cross the corpus callosum from the left to the right hemisphere. The col-

onel's callosal lesion interfered with the transfer of motor knowledge, and not spelling knowledge, because the cyst was located in
the anterior portion of the corpus callosum.

The memories of how to move the hand to form letters and the
knowledge of how words are spelled cross the corpus callosum at
different areas. From studying patients such as Colonel Thomas, we
believe that motor knowledge crosses anteriorly and spelling knowledge posteriorly.

We have discussed the colonel's deficits in detail because he
demonstrates that there are at least two major types of agraphia:
apraxic (loss of motor skills) and linguistic.

Apraxic Agraphia: Inability to Form Letters

Although in most people the left hemisphere contains both the
memories of how words are spelled and the movements needed to
form letters, occasionally dissociation occurs. About 25 years ago, I
examined a left-handed man who, as a boy, started writing with his
left hand but was forced by his teachers to use his right hand. When
as an adult he had a stroke that affected his right hemisphere, causing weakness of his left arm, he lost the ability to write with his right
hand—the hand he had written with for many decades, but when
given a typewriter, he was able to type correctly. It appears that
although this man wrote with his right hand, it was still his right
hemisphere that stored the memories of how to move to produce
letters. The stroke had destroyed these memories. Unlike the letter
movement memories, the memories, or representations, of how the
words are spelled appeared to be stored in his left hemisphere, and
when provided with a typewriter, he did not have to form the letters
and therefore could type.

In assessing this man's ability to make skilled, learned movements, we tested not only his writing, but also his ability to perform
other skills, such as using a pair of scissors or a screwdriver. We found
that he was also impaired in making these movements, suggesting
that the memories, or representations, of these movements had also
been destroyed. That this man had lost the knowledge both of how
to form letters and how to perform skilled movements suggests that
perhaps there is only one storage area for all motor skills. David
Roeltgen and I, however, have seen patients who lost the knowledge
of how to form letters but could perform other skilled movements.

We have also examined patients who lost the ability to use tools correctly but could still write letters normally, suggesting that the representations of the movements used to write are stored separately from the knowledge of how to use tools and make other skilled movements.

Linguistic Agraphia: A Loss of Spelling Knowledge

When we discussed reading disorders, we explained that there are two ways to read words. One can transform letters into the sounds these letters represent (grapheme-to-phoneme) or one can use a whole-word (lexical) approach. When writing, there are also two methods that can be used to select the letters needed to write a word. One can break the word into its component speech sounds, or phonemes, and find the letters (graphemes) that represent these speech sounds or one can use a whole word (lexical) approach.

The inability to changes speech sounds into letters is called *phonological agraphia* and the inability to use the whole-word method of writing is called *lexical agraphia*. Patients with phonological agraphia will have difficulty writing words to which they have not been repeatedly exposed. They may have the most difficulty writing nonwords such as *flig*. Because they must rely on the lexical or whole-word system, they may spell *flig* as *flag*. In contrast, patients with lexical agraphia should be able to write most regular words, like *dog* or *cat*, but may have trouble writing words like *comb*. If their lexical representations of words like *comb* are gone, they will use the grapheme-to-phoneme system and may spell the word *kome*. In English a final *e* usually makes the preceding vowel (the *o*) a long sound or the sound of the letter. Therefore, when asked to spell the word *come*, they will spell it *cum* or *kum*.

Patients with lexical agraphia usually have lesions in their dominant, or left-sided, poster parietal lobe, primarily in the region of the angular gyrus (Fig. 2–12). In contrast, most of the patients with phonological agraphia we have studied had lesions in a more anterior portion of the inferior parietal lobe, mainly in the anterior supramarginal gyrus (Fig. 2–12). Therefore, the angular gyrus must contain the memories of how words are spelled, and the supramarginal gyrus must have the ability to convert speech sounds into letters.

Many patients have a combined deficit, so that they are unable

Summary

There are two major elements to writing: linguistic and praxic. The linguistic element allows us to spell words, and the praxic element allows us to program the movements needed to form letters. There are two methods of spelling. One can use the whole-word (lexical) process or translate each word sound (phoneme) into the letters that symbolize this sound. In order to select the correct word to write, the meaning or the semantic–conceptual system must influence the word choice. In right-handed people, these praxic and linguistic writing systems are mediated by the left hemisphere. This writing system is parallel to and independent of the reading and speech systems but also interacts with them. The writing system we have discussed is summarized diagrammatically in Figure 2–15.

Selected Readings

Beauvois, M.F., Derouesne, J. (1981) Lexical or orthographic agraphia. *Brain* 104:21–49.

Benson, D.F. (1979) *Aphasia, alexia, agraphia*, Churchill Livingston, New York.

McCarthy, R.A., Warrington, E.K., (1990) Spelling and writing. In *Cognitive neuropsychology*. Academic Press, New York, pp. 241–261.

Roeltgen, D.P. (1993) Agraphia. In *Clinical Neuropsychology*. (ed.) Heilman, K.M., and Valenstein, E., Oxford University Press, New York, pp. 63–89.

Roeltgen, D.P., Heilman, K.M., (1985) Review of agraphia and proposal for an anatomically based model. *Appl. Psycholinguistics* 6: 205–230.

Shallice, T. (1981) Phonological agraphia and the lexical route in writing. *Brain* 104:412–429.

3

EMOTIONS

In this chapter, we will consider two subjects in the study of emotion. The first subject is how people convey their own emotions and understand the emotions of others, and how these processes are disturbed with injury to the brain. The second subject is how we experience emotion and how this experience, and the behavior that flows from it, are altered by brain injury.

EMOTIONAL COMMUNICATION

Speech Prosody

The person who sparked my interest in disorders of emotional communication was Paula Robins, a 46-year-old housewife and mother of two. In the summer of 1971 a family physician in Orlando called me about her. After 3 days of headaches, she had suffered a series seizures and was now comatose. The physician was not sure what was happening to Mrs. Robins or how to treat her. He had given her Ativan, an anticonvulsant, that appeared to stop the seizures, but she was still comatose. He and her husband wanted to transfer her to the Shands Teaching Hospital at the University of Florida. She arrived in our emergency room about 2 hours after his call. Her vital signs were normal except for a slight fever. Because there is always a risk of hypoglycemia (low blood sugar) causing coma and seizures, we routinely give patients glucose. We also started giving her the anticonvulsant Dilantin. She was comatose but did respond to painful stimuli. One way we induce painful stimulation is to rub the sternum (breastbone). When doing this, I noticed that while the patient moved her arms toward her breastbone, her right arm moved more than her left arm. Similarly, when I scratched the bottom of her feet, she moved the right leg more than the left. These motor signs suggested that her right hemisphere was damaged. This suspicion was confirmed when I tested her reflexes and found that they were abnormal on the left side. In addition, her eyes tended to deviate toward the right. Each hemisphere of the brain not only controls the opposite side of the body but is also responsible for moving the eyes in the opposite direction. Because Mrs. Robins kept looking to the right, her right hemisphere appeared to be injured, so that she could not move her eyes to the left. Unfortunately, when we first saw her, CT or MRI brain imaging was not available. Because she had seizures, a low-grade fever, and evidence of right hemisphere brain damage, I was concerned that there might be an infection in the right hemisphere. To find out, we decided to perform a lumbar puncture (spinal tap). Her spinal fluid showed an increased number of white blood cells and an elevated protein level, suggesting an infection. We did not see any bacteria and no bacteria grew on culture, which indicated that the condition was not bacterial meningitis. Based on these findings, we diagnosed a focal brain infection. We could not be sure if it was viral or bacterial, but since there was no treatment for viral infections at that time, we treated her with antibiotics for a possible bacterial infection. We did obtain an EEG, which showed an epileptic focus in her right parietal lobe consistent with a focal infection or abscess. A radioisotope scan also showed abnormal activity over this parietal area consistent with an abscess. With antibiotic and anticonvulsant treatment, Mrs. Robins slowly improved. She became more alert. Her left-sided weakness and left-sided gaze disorder also improved. Before discharge from the hospital, the only sign she showed was a neglect of left space, being unaware of people and things located on the left side of her body. She went home with a prescription for Dilantin.

Because Mrs. Robins had a left-sided neglect syndrome, I told her and her husband that she should not drive. Three months after her discharge, Mr. Robins brought her to the clinic. She was doing well. She had no seizures and was taking Dilantin regularly, and her blood level of this anticonvulsant was within the therapeutic range. Her husband told me that although she missed some things on her left side, she was now doing some cooking and cleaning. Because Mrs. Robins continued demonstrating signs of left-sided neglect, I again suggested that she not drive. I renewed her prescription for Dilantin and asked the Robinses to return to the clinic in 6 months.

Six months later, Mrs. Robins was doing even better. She remained on Dilantin and had had no further seizures. Her blood level of Dilantin was still in the therapeutic range, and her physical examination was normal except for a very mild degree of left-sided neglect. While she was putting on her shoes, her husband signaled that he wanted to talk to me privately. We found an empty room, and Mr. Robins asked, "If I left my wife, would she be able to make it by herself?" My impression had been that Mr. Robins was very fond of his wife and very concerned about losing her when she was sick. I did not understand why now, when she was getting better, he wanted to leave her.

Unfortunately, I have the wrong personality to be a psychiatrist or clinical psychologist. In medical school I was taught nondirective therapy, in which the clinician listens passively to patients when they discuss their problems. My family and friends have often noted that being nondirective is not part of my personality. Thus, rather then listen passively to him, I asked, "What about the children?" He said that both of them had already left home to go to college. Then I asked, "Do you have a new girlfriend?" He said, "No, that's not why I want to leave her." He went on to tell me that they no longer had a "meaningful relationship." Unsure of what he meant, I asked, "What do you mean? She is your wife." He looked uncomfortable, squirmed in his chair, and said, "Before coming to Florida, I worked for a tire company in Dayton for 20 years. During that time I saved money because my dream was to move to Florida and open my own store. I opened a store in Orlando not far from Disney World. It was mainly a tee shirt and souvenir shop. The first year I almost broke even, which is not bad for a new business, but this year has been devastating." A recession had occurred, along with a national gasoline shortage and high inflation. Fewer tourists came to Florida, and those who did come spent less money. His business was hard hit. He said, "I'm almost bankrupt." His voice started to quiver. "I've been terribly upset about this. When I come home there is sadness written all over my face, and when I speak I sound sad and depressed, but my wife never recognizes that anything is wrong. If a wife is insensitive to her husband's emotions, how can they have a meaningful relationship?"

People who have meaningful relationships sometimes say, "It is not what you said, but how you said it that counts." The "how you said it" element is called *speech prosody*. When we speak, in addition to producing the sounds that constitute words, we change the pitch, loudness, overtones (timbre), and speed of our voice. Brenda Milner, a famous neuropsychologist at the Montreal Neurological Institute, had studied patients who had sections of either the right or left side of their brain removed because their epilepsy could not be controlled by anticonvulsant medications. She was interested in learning which hemisphere was dominant for appreciating music. She found that each hemisphere plays a different role. For example, the left hemisphere is important for recognizing rhythms and the right for recognizing melody and timbre. Because melody and timbre recognition is mediated by the right hemisphere, I had begun to think that the right hemisphere might also be important for understanding not what is said but how it is said. I told Mr. Robins, "Let's go back to the room. I want to give your wife some tests." When we returned, I said to Mrs. Robins, "I'm going to say a sentence. Please listen to my speech, and based on the tone of my voice and not the words I am saying, tell me how I feel." I then said, "Fish can jump out of the sea." I spoke the sentence with emotional prosody that indicated sadness. After listening to this sentence Mrs. Robins said, "You're happy." I asked her why she thought so. She said, "Watching fish jump out of the sea would make me happy." Again I explained what I wanted her to do. "Listen to how I say the sentence, not to what I say." Then I spoke more sentences with emotional prosody. Her responses were almost random. Although she was college educated and extremely intelligent, she could not understand emotional prosody. Observing this, her husband realized that he would have to explain his emotions to her verbally. Unfortunately, his store did fail, he became bankrupt, and they moved back to Ohio. I never learned whether he succeeded in repairing their relationship.

After examining Mrs. Robins, I searched the scientific and clinical literature for reports of what happened to emotional prosody with brain damage. When I found none, my colleagues and I decided to study patients with left and right hemisphere lesions to learn if the right hemisphere is indeed dominant for understanding emotional prosody. We found that although patients with left hemisphere strokes were often aphasic, they performed almost flawlessly when asked to identify the emotions communicated in sentences that were intoned with emotional prosody. Patients with right hemisphere damage, however, performed very poorly. This study was performed before neuroimaging existed, so we could not be certain where in the right hemisphere the damage had occurred. However, based on the patients' signs and symptoms, we thought that their strokes had destroyed the right inferior parietal lobe and the right posterior temporal lobe (Fig. 3–1).

The right and left hemispheres are connected by the corpus callosum, a large group of nerves that go from one side of the cerebral cortex to the other. The corpus callosum is an important part of the brain because it lets one hemisphere know what the other knows or is doing. If you give a blindfolded patient whose corpus

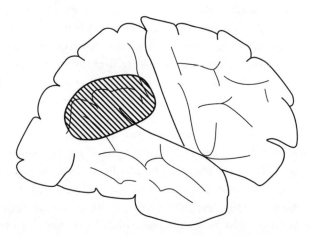

Figure 3–1. Diagram of a right hemisphere injury that interferes with the ability to understand the emotional prosody expressed in speech.

callosum is damaged (from a stroke or neurosurgery for seizures) objects to feel in the right hand, she or he will be able to name the objects. Information from the right hand goes to the sensory cortex in the left hemisphere. From here, this information goes to a tactile association area and then to the language areas where the object is named. If, however, you ask this blindfolded patient to name an object that you have placed in his or her left hand, the patient will be unable to name it. Sensory systems from the left side of the body project to the right hemisphere's sensory cortex and then to sensory association areas. To gain access to the language-speech areas, this information has to be transmitted from the right hemisphere's senory association areas to the left hemisphere's language areas. If the corpus callosum has been severed, the sensory information from the right hemisphere cannot be transmitted to the left hemisphere's language areas. Although blindfolded patients with callosal section cannot name objects by feeling them with the left hand, if you let them feel two different objects or two of the same objects with the left hand, they will have no difficulty indicating that the two objects are the same or different because the left hemisphere language areas are not required for this determination.

The patients who could not tell our examiners the emotional states associated with emotional speech intonation or prosody had right hemisphere lesions. We knew it was possible that these lesions had disconnected the right hemisphere from the left and that the patients were unable to identify the emotional prosody of speech because this prosodic information could not reach the language-speech areas in the left hemisphere. To test this hypothesis, we studied another group of patients with either right or left hemisphere strokes, but this time, rather than asking them to name the emotion, we presented two different sentences that were intoned with emotion. In half of the trials the emotional prosody of the two sentences was the same; in the other half, it was different. We randomized the order in which the same and different trials were given. We asked the patients to tell us if the emotional tone of the two sentences was the same or different. The left hemisphere aphasic patients performed this task almost flawlessly, but the patients with right hemisphere damage performed very poorly. These results suggest that the patients with right hemisphere strokes were making errors not because they failed to find the names for the expressed emotional intonations, but because another problem(s) accounted for this deficit.

In English we distinguish words from one another by the phonemes that form them. For example, the difference in the words *bat* and *hat* is between the *b* and *h* sounds. In some Asian languages, two words with the same phonemes can have different meanings if they are spoken with different intonations or prosody. In English, prosody does not change the meaning of words, but we do use prosody for syntactic or grammatical reasons. For example, if you say "The boy took the bus" and drop the tone of your voice at the end of the sentence, it tells the listener that this is a statement or a declarative sentence. If you speak the same words but raise the tone of your voice at the end, it becomes a question or interrogative sentence. In contrast to the emotional prosody we discussed earlier, we will call this *grammatical prosody*. Sandra Weintraub and Marcel Mesulam wanted to learn if the prosodic defects we described were limited to emotional prosody or included the grammatical type as well. They tested patients with right hemisphere strokes and normal controls for their comprehension of grammatical prosody. Compared to control subjects, the patients with right hemisphere strokes had trouble understanding grammatical prosody. Weintraub and Mesulam concluded that the right hemisphere is dominant for comprehending prosody independent of whether the prosody is emotional or nonemotional. Unfortunately, this conclusion may have been premature. In the Asian languages, where prosody can change the meaning of words, left rather than right hemisphere damage impairs understanding of this form of prosody. Weintraub and Mesulam did not compare patients with right hemisphere strokes to those with left hemisphere strokes. Nor did they did not compare grammatical prosody to emotional prosody. We compared right–and left hemisphere–damaged patients for the comprehension of both emotional and grammatical prosody and found that Weintraub and Mesulam were correct: right hemisphere damage does interfere with the comprehension of grammatical prosody. We also found, however, that left hemisphere injury interferes with the comprehension of grammatical prosody. In addition, right hemisphere damage interrupts the comprehension of emotional prosody more than left hemisphere damage does, suggesting that the right hemisphere is dominant for comprehending emotional but not grammatical prosody.

Although these experiments suggested that the right hemisphere is dominant for understanding prosody, there is another possible explanation of these results. Dawn Bowers and I studied hemispheric attentional asymmetries while she was a graduate student in the 1970s. When a person attempts to listen to a specific auditory stimulus in the presence of other sounds, he or she must distinguish the target sounds from the nontarget sounds (noise) and filter out the noise. We wanted to learn whether one hemisphere that is specialized to deal with certain stimuli, such as language or music, does a better job of filtering out these stimuli when they represent noise or is more distracted by stimuli that it is specialized to process. As discussed above, the right hemisphere is dominant in recognizing melodies and the left in comprehending speech. Each ear is more strongly connected to the opposite hemisphere. We gave normal subjects the task of recognizing music when someone was speaking or recognizing speech when background music was playing. When subjects were trying to listen to speech, the left ear–right hemisphere was more distracted by music, and when they were trying to listen to music, the right–ear left hemisphere was more distracted by speech. Thus, each hemisphere is more distracted by stimuli it ordinarily processes.

When we had presented emotionally intoned sentences to patients, the prosody was superimposed on emotionally neutral sentences. Could it be that the left hemisphere had the potential to understand emotional prosody but was being distracted by listening selectively to the words in the sentences? To test this possibility, we again studied patients who had suffered right hemisphere strokes by giving them sentences spoken with emotional prosody. If these patients were being distracted when the verbal content of the sentences conflicted with the prosody, they should have performed more poorly than when the content was neutral. For example, if we said, "My dog just died" with a happy tone, they should have had more trouble recognizing the prosody than if we spoke a neutral sentence such as "The boy went up the stairs" with a happy tone. That is exactly what we found. The study revealed that in right hemisphere–damaged patients, the normal left hemisphere was being distracted by the verbal content of the sentence. This result suggests that the left hemisphere may be able to comprehend emotional prosody but can be distracted by the meaning of words. It is also possible that whereas the left hemisphere does have some capacity to comprehend prosody, the right hemisphere is still dominant. To test this hypothesis further, we again gave patients emotionally intoned sentences but filtered out the high-frequency speech sounds. This filtering procedure does not affect the comprehension of prosody in normal people, but it makes the verbal message, incomprehensible. Since there no verbal message, the left hemisphere will not be distracted. The right hemisphere–damaged patients were still more impaired than those with left hemisphere injuries, providing further evidence that the right hemisphere is dominant for the comprehension of emotional prosody.

Some critics of our studies suggested that the aphasic patients with left hemisphere damage to whom we compared our right hemisphere–damaged patients did not have severe left hemisphere injuries because most of them were able to comprehend words. Recently, Anna Barrett and I saw a 34-year-old woman, Cathy Henson, who had been healthy all her life. On the day of admission to the hospital, she suddenly developed paralysis of her right arm and leg and became unable to speak, to understand speech or writing, or to name and repeat. This syndrome, called *global aphasia*, usually indicates a very large left hemisphere injury that has destroyed the entire language cortex. Why a young woman with no risk factors would have a massive stoke was unclear. When an MRI scan was performed, it confirmed our clinical impression. Much of her left hemisphere had been destroyed. A study of the blood vessels leading to the brain revealed that one of the major arteries, the left carotid, had a tear, or dissection. When a vessel tears, clots form on the inside of the vessel wall. These clots can prevent blood from reaching the brain or can break off and clog other vessels that feed blood to the brain.

Mrs. Henson was treated with anticoagulants to prevent more clots from forming. We kept her in the hospital to regulate her medication. One day we were in her hospital room when her husband and three children came to visit. It was apparent that she adored her family and they loved her. It was also apparent that although she could not understand what they were saying, she did seem to appreciate their vocal emotional expressions. We decided to test Cathy to see if we could demonstrate that she understood emotional prosody. When we presented tape recordings of an actress speaking sentences with emotional intonations, Cathy could not name the emotion expressed. We then showed her pictures of a person making a sad, happy, angry, or neutral face and gestured to indicate that she should point to the appropriate face. She immediately understood the task and performed it almost flawlessly. She also had no difficulty discriminating between two spoken sentences that had different emotional prosody. These observations provided additional evidence that the right hemisphere is important for understanding emotional prosody.

As mentioned before, the nerves from each ear project to the opposite hemisphere more than to the hemisphere on the same side. If you simultaneously present normal subjects with two intoned words, one to each ear, and ask which word they heard, they are more likely to report the word that they heard with their right ear. But if you ask them the emotional tone of the words, they are more likely to identify the prosody presented to the left ear–right hemisphere.

Several clinicians, such as Guido Gainotti and his colleagues, observed that patients with right hemisphere damage from strokes appear to be emotionally indifferent. Because we had found that patients with right hemisphere strokes had problems comprehending emotional prosody, we wondered if there were patients with right hemisphere damage who also had problems expressing emotional prosody. We tested patients with right hemisphere disease by asking them to repeat neutral-content sentences (e.g., "The boy walked to the store") with emotional prosody (e.g., sadness). We recorded their speech and played the tapes to trained judges who were unaware of the clinical status of the subjects (e.g., patients with right hemisphere injury or control subjects) and the emotion the subjects were trying to express. When the judges listened to these tapes, they thought that unlike the control subjects' sentences, most of the sentences spoken by the right hemisphere–damaged patients were neutral or indifferent. These results suggested that patients with right hemisphere injuries were impaired not only in comprehending emotional prosody but also in expressing it.

When we tested our first subject with right hemisphere damage for the ability to express emotional prosody, we asked him to repeat the sentence "The boy went to the store" with a sad intonation. He said, "The boy went to the store. He was sad." Because we did not want the judges to know the target emotion, we told the patient, "Please, don't say that he was sad. Instead, just say 'The boy went to the store' and make the tone of you voice sound sad." The patient then said, "The sad boy went to the store." Since we could not persuade the right hemisphere–damaged patients to stop using this verbal strategy, we had to edit our tapes so that the judges would remain unaware of the target prosody. Because the patients with right hemisphere injuries could not express emotional intonations in their sentences, they may have been using a verbal strategy to overcome their disability. These patients are the opposite of the nonfluent aphasics discussed in the "Speech" section, Chapter 2, who, being unable to produce fluent speech, often say one or two words with a variety of emotional intonations.

After we reported that patients with right hemisphere injuries often cannot understand and express emotional prosody, Elliot Ross and Marcel Mesulam also described two patients who were unable to express emotional prosody. Unlike our patients, however, they could comprehend emotional prosody. Both of these patients had right hemisphere lesions located primarily in the frontal lobes. Elliot Ross later hypothesized that emotional prosody is organized in the right hemisphere similarly to the way propositional speech is organized in the left hemisphere. The posterior (e.g., temporal and parietal) region is important for comprehension, and the anterior (e.g., right frontal lobe) region is important for expression.

Facial Expressions

When one is experiencing an emotion or a mood, this may be expressed not only vocally but also facially. When Paula Robins (the patient from Orlando who had the right parietal abscess) was unaware of her husband's sad mood, perhaps she could not recognize both his sad emotional speech prosody and his sad face. Since the right temporal parietal region is important for comprehending emotional prosody, it may also be important for understanding emotional facial expressions. To test this theory, we photographed people expressing four different emotions (happy, sad, angry, and neutral) facially. We then asked a group of patients with left and right hemisphere damage from strokes either to name the emotional facial expression in these photos or to point to one of four photographed faces expressing the emotion named by the examiner. We also showed the subjects pictures of two faces and asked them whether the faces were expressing the same emotion or different emotions. Compared to patients with left hemisphere disease, those with right hemisphere disease had trouble naming facial emotional expressions, pointing to faces expressing emotions named by the examiner, and telling if two faces were expressing the same emotion or different emotions.

Dawn Bowers and I saw a man who could not correctly name the emotions displayed on faces. For example, if we showed him a picture of an actor portraying anger and asked him to name the emotion, he might say, "Happy." This man was not aphasic and had no problem naming objects. Because we wanted to learn if his deficit was specific for naming emotions rather than a general inability to recognize facial emotional expressions, we showed him a series of pictures of actors displaying four different emotions and asked him to point to (rather than name) the face expressing the emotion named by the examiner. He also performed this task poorly, often pointing to the incorrect face. But when shown a series of cards, each containing two pictures of actors' faces displaying the same emotion or different emotions, and asked if the two faces displayed the same emotion or different emotions, his performance was flawless. He could also match emotional prosody with facial emotional expressions. A CT scan revealed that this man had a tumor deep in his right hemisphere. The tumor interrupted the nerve fibers going to and coming from the corpus callosum that normally carry information between the two hemispheres. Because language, including the ability to name emotions, is mediated by the left hemisphere and the recognition of facial emotional expressions is mediated by the right hemisphere, this tumor dissociated these functions by disconnecting the two hemispheres.

After completing these facial emotion comprehension studies, we tried to determine if there were hemispheric asymmetries in the control of emotional facial expressions. We photographed right–and left hemisphere–injured patients while they were attempting to make these faces and then showed the photographs to judges who knew neither the clinical history of these patients or which emotion they were trying to express. There was no difference in the ability of right–and left hemisphere–damaged patients to express facial emotions. However, no matter how well one designs an experiment, methodological problems almost always occur. For example, if we had recorded videos rather than still photographs, we might have seen hemispheric asymmetries, or if we had photographed true emotional responses rather than posed expressions, differences might have emerged. Although we considered reporting our negative results, we were concerned about such methodological problems and decided not to submit the report. Later, Lee Blonder recorded videotapes of patients who were actually experiencing an emotion and found that the patients with right hemisphere injury were indeed impaired in expressing facial emotions. Other investigators reported similar results.

These studies of patients with discrete brain injuries suggest that the right hemisphere is normally important for comprehending and expressing facial emotions. This is, however, only an inference, and it would be helpful to have converging evidence from tests of normal people. Support for the hypothesis that normally the right hemisphere is important for comprehending and expressing facial emotion comes from studies of normal subjects. If you look straight ahead and an image is flashed to your left side, this image will be carried to the right hemisphere. Similarly, if an image is flashed to your right side, it will travel to the left hemisphere. Using this experimental approach, researchers found that when images of emotional faces were flashed to either the right or the left hemisphere, normal subjects recognized the emotional expressions better when they were flashed to the left side (right hemisphere) than when they were flashed to the right side (left hemisphere).

To learn if there are asymmetries of emotional expression in normal people, Harold Sackheim took the negatives of photographs of normal subjects expressing emotions facially and cut them vertically in half through the nose so that one eye was on one side of the cut and the other eye was on the other side. He then duplicated both the right and left half negatives, turned one half around, and fused this inverted image with the other half so that there now appeared to be a full face composed of either two left or two right half faces. He showed these combined left and right faces to judges and asked them to rate the strength of the emotion that the images expressed. On average, the judges thought that the images made from the left side of faces had stronger emotional expressions than those made from the right side. Since the left side of the brain controls the right side of the face, and vice versa, these results support the hypothesis that the right hemisphere primarily controls the facial expression of emotion.

While it is clear that the right hemisphere plays a dominant role in both the comprehension and expression of nonverbal emotional signals, the brain mechanisms underlying these functions are more difficult to ascertain. As I discussed in the "Speech" section of Chapter 2, there are at least three levels of analysis for the comprehension of words in the left hemisphere. When we listen to speech, the brain performs an auditory analysis, activates phonological lexical representations (memories of word sounds), and finally activates the semantic–conceptual network to derive the meaning of the lexical representation. Perhaps the comprehension of facial emotional expressions and emotional prosody also requires three levels of analysis: sensory analysis, activation of the images of prototypic emotional faces or prototypic emotional prosody, and activation of emotional semantics. To determine at what level(s) patients with right hemisphere disease are impaired in the understanding of emotion, Lee Blonder and other investigators in our laboratory studied a group of patients who had trouble identifying emotional facial expressions by asking them to listen to two types of sentences. One type described emotional gestures (e.g., "Tears came to his eyes"), and the other type described situations that would induce an emotion (e.g., "The kids tracked mud all over her new white carpet"). These sentences were generated by a computer because we wanted to avoid emotional prosody and because we were concerned that if actors read the sentences into a tape recorder, they would automatically add prosody. After these right hemisphere–damaged patients and normal subjects heard a sentence, they were asked to tell the examiner what kind of emotion the person in such a situation might be experiencing. Compared to the normal subjects, the right hemisphere–damaged patients had difficulty comprehending the verbal descriptions of emotional gestures. But they performed just as well as normal controls when we presented sentences describing situations and asked them to infer the emotion they would feel in those situations. These results suggest that right hemisphere damage does not impair emotional semantics. Because many of the patients had large right hemisphere lesions, the results indicate that the left as well as the right hemisphere can mediate emotional semantics. Even when vision and the perception of spatial relations were not involved, the patients with right hemisphere lesions had trouble recognizing descriptions of emotional faces. This indicates that the memories, or representations, of prototypical emotional faces in these patients were either destroyed or inaccessible.

To further explore this issue, Dawn Bowers and others in our laboratory asked right–and left hemisphere–damaged patients and normal control subjects questions about either objects (e.g., "Where is the year printed on a penny?") or emotional faces (e.g., "What emotion is associated with dilation of the nostrils"?) To carry out this task, most people will image the object or the emotional facial expression. We found that the left hemisphere–damaged patients had difficulty imaging objects but not emotional faces. In contrast, the right hemisphere–damaged patients imaged emotional faces poorly but did well with objects. Because patients with right hemisphere strokes could image objects in a normal fashion, their problem with imaging emotional faces could not be explained by an overall deficit in imaging. Imaging an emotional face depends on having a memory of what that kind of face looks like. If right hemisphere damage had either destroyed the facial emotional representations or interfered with their activation, then the patients should not have been able to recognize the emotions expressed by the faces, should not have recognized descriptions of emotional faces, and should not have been able to image emotional faces. Patients with right temporal-parietal damage performed all of these tasks poorly.

Although injury to the right posterior temporal-parietal region impairs the recognition of both emotional faces and speech prosody, some patients cannot comprehend emotional prosody but can recognize emotional faces, while other patients show the reverse pattern. This dissociation suggests that the neural representations for emotional prosody and faces are independent.

Paul Ekman took photographs of actors making emotional faces. He showed these photographs to people all over the world, including people from primitive cultures where movies and television were not available. Wherever he went, about seven of the same basic emotional expressions were recognized by people of all races and cultures (i.e., happiness, sadness, anger, fear, surprise, disgust, boredom). The words used to express these emotions are not universally recognized. This dissociation suggests that words but not emotional faces are learned. Because facial emotions are universal, their neural representations are probably genetically programmed. Further evidence supporting this theory comes from the observation that even young infants can recognize emotions expressed on their mother's face. Although not tested, we suspect that emotional prosody of speech is not entirely learned but is also genetically programmed. But how would it be programmed? If I asked you, "In what direction do you turn a screwdriver to take out a screw?" before you answered "Counterclockwise" you might feel your arm attempt to turn the screw. Although we initially thought that emotional facial representations are iconic (information stored in picture form), they might be stored as motor programs similar to that of using a screwdriver. Patients with Parkinson's disease often have immobile faces. To learn if knowledge about emotional facial expressions might be stored in movement programs, we asked a group of patients with Parkinson's disease to recognize and image emotional faces. They had trouble doing so. This observation provides evidence that the representations of facial emotions may be stored as motor programs; we are continuing to test this hypothesis.

In the "Speech" section of Chapter 2, we provided evidence that the left hemisphere mediates propositional language, and in this chapter we have provided evidence that the right brain mediates emotional communication. Are there advantages to this design? We do not have the answer, but one advantage might be that this arrangement allows parallel processing. Thus, when listening to someone with whom you have a meaningful relationship, you can simultaneously hear and understand not only what is said (cognitively), but also how it is said (emotionally).

Summary

Speech can simultaneously carry two messages, propositional (statements) and emotional. The propositional message is communicated by the use of words. Although the emotional message may also be carried by words, it is often conveyed by changes in the tone of voice, or prosody. Studies of patients with brain damage suggest that whereas the left hemisphere is important for expressing and comprehending propositional speech, the right hemisphere mediates the comprehension and expression of emotional prosody. In the right hemisphere, the right posterior temporal and parietal lobes are important for comprehension and the right frontal lobe is important for the expression of emotional prosody. Having the left hemisphere mediate propositional speech while the right hemisphere mediates emotional prosody allows a person to perform parallel processes, and to hear or express both a propositional and a prosodic emotional message simultaneously.

Facial expressions are also used to communicate emotions. Studies of brain-damaged patients suggest that the right hemisphere is dominant for the comprehension and expression of emotional faces, the right posterior temporal-parietal region being important for comprehension, and the right frontal lobe for expression. Although interactive, the representations of emotional prosody and emotional faces are independent. Whereas the words used to express ideas are learned, emotional expressions are universal, suggesting that the facial movements and prosody used to express emotions are inborn. Perhaps that is why even young infants can recognize emotional facial expressions and emotional prosody.

EMOTIONAL EXPERIENCE

Humans can experience a variety of primary emotions such as happiness, sadness, fear, anger, surprise, boredom, and disgust. These emotional experiences have profound effects on behavior both when the person is experiencing the emotion and after the experience is over. For example, anger may lead us to approach the object that induced our anger, and fear may lead us to avoid the object that caused it. Even when we are not feeling an emotion, we seek the stimuli and situations that make us joyous and avoid those that make us sad.

It was once thought that the heart was the organ of emotion, but Hippocrates (ca. 460–377 B.C.E.) contended that "One ought to know that the brain, and from the brain only, arise our pleasures, joys, laughter and jests, as well as our sorrows, pains, griefs and tears." Almost everyone now agrees that the brain is the organ of emotions, but the underlying mechanisms remain unclear. Much of what we know about the human neurobiology of emotions comes from observing brain-damaged patients. In this section we will explore some of the major theories that have been proposed to explain emotional experience.

Feedback Theories

According to one group of theories, emotional feelings, like other sensations, come from feedback to the brain. After the brain interprets stimuli, it activates organs such as the heart and skeletal muscles, including those of the face. For example, if we see something frightening, like a person approaching with a knife, the brain inter-

prets this visual stimulus as a threat to our lives and sends a message
for the heart to beat faster and the face to expresses fear, with the
eyes becoming wider and the mouth opening. Charles Darwin, at
the end of the nineteenth century, was probably the first to describe
the facial feedback theory when he suggested that the free expression of outward signs of an emotion intensifies it and the repression
of all outward signs weakens it. The facial feedback theory posits
that when the brain detects changes in the face, the person experiences emotional feelings. This theory might account for the British
saying, when they desire emotional restraint, "Keep a stiff upper lip."
Walter Cannon suggested that these changes serve adaptive pur-
poses. For example, a more rapid heartbeat might help us run or
fight, and an opening mouth might allow more air to enter our
lungs.

Recently, a college student, Sarah Smith, helped us provide evidence against the facial feedback theory. Sarah was a very talented
athlete who played guard on the women's basketball team at the
University of Florida. It was her senior year, and the Gators had a
chance to win the South Eastern Conference championship and perhaps even the national championship. Sarah also had a chance to
be drafted by the newly formed women's professional basketball association. Learning that a flu epidemic might be coming to Gainesville, she decided to be vaccinated. Several weeks after the vaccination, during practice for the season's first game, she noticed that she
was running a little more slowly and could not jump as high as usual.
She also realized that athletes have bad days and thought that this
might be one of them. The next day, however, she could hardly run,
and when she tried to jump, her feet hardly left the floor. Her coach
also noticed these problems, and they decided to go to the hospital
emergency room. Sarah was seen by one of our residents, who found
that her legs were weak and that she had lost her deep tendon reflexes. When he hit the tendon below the knee cap, for example,
her leg did not jerk forward, as it does in normal people. He diagnosed her condition as Guillain-Barré-syndrome, or acute postinfec-
tious polyneuritis, a possible complication of flu vaccination. In this
disease, the person's immune system produces antibodies against the
nerves that travel from the spinal cord and brain stem to the muscles
of the body and face. These antibodies interfere with nerve function,
leading to weakness and a loss of reflexes. The neuropathy usually
starts in the legs and progresses up the body. In the most dangerous

situation, the immune system attacks the nerves traveling to the muscles that are important for breathing. Sarah was treated with intravenous administration of antibodies that reduced her production of abnormal antibodies. She never lost her ability to breathe and did not have to be put on a respirator, but despite the treatment her face became totally paralyzed. She could swallow but not chew and thus did not need to be fed through a tube. However, when she was fed, her mouth had to be opened. Her facial weakness was so severe that she could not speak or even blink her eyes, and there was no detectable movement of any facial muscle. She did, however, maintain a little strength in her arms, and her friend made her two personas, or masks; one showed sadness and the other happiness. When she wanted to express one of these two emotions, she held up the appropriate mask. During the period when her face was paralyzed, Jocelyn Kiellor and Anna Barrett tested her ability to experience emotions by showing her slides of pictures that evoke emotions in normal college students, including pictures of people with bloody, mutilated bodies. After presenting each slide, they asked Sarah to indicate, by pointing to a series of cartoons, how the slide made her feel. Although she could not move a single muscle of her face, Sarah's emotional responses were completely normal. These results indicate that sensory feedback from the face is not important for emotional experience.

The visceral feedback theory (e.g., feedback from the heart to the brain) was first put forth at the close of the nineteenth century by the founder of modern psychology, William James. About 25 years later, Gregorio Marañon injected epinephrine into people and asked them what emotion they were experiencing. Epinephrine is the hormone produced when we experience negative emotions such as fear and anger. During these emotional experiences the heart often beats faster, and when people are given epinephrine the heart rate also increases. Marañon's subjects said that they felt "as if" they should be feeling an emotion, but they were not actually experiencing one. These observations provide evidence against the visceral feedback theory. Stanley Schacter, however, thought that these subjects did not experience an emotion because nothing was happening to them to which they could attribute the increased heartbeat induced by epinephrine. Experiencing an emotion, according to Schacter, requires two basic elements: visceral arousal and an environmental situation to which one can attribute the visceral change.

To test his hypothesis, he injected epinephrine into one group of students who had agreed to participate in a vision experiment. Another group of students who were not injected served as control subjects. Students who had to wait before having their vision tested were placed in a room with an actor and were asked to perform activities designed to make them angry or happy. The students reported their experiences, and there were also raters who did not know whether a subject had been injected with epinephrine. Subjects who had received epinephrine but were not placed in the room with the actor had the same "as if" feelings described by Marañon. Those who had not received epinephrine but were placed with the actor did feel some emotions, but these emotions were not very strong. Those who had received the epinephrine and were also placed with the actor felt strong emotions and were also judged by the raters to have the strongest emotions. The results of this classic experiment seem to support Schacter's attribution-arousal feedback theory of emotional experience.

Inconsistent with Schacter's theory are my observations of a 19-year-old Northeastern University epileptic college student named Portia. Although she was reluctant to admit it, during some of her seizures, in addition to shaking all over, she had urinated on herself and had even bitten her tongue. After the seizures ended, Portia was sleepy and confused for about an hour. The type of seizure she described was then known as a *grand mal* (big bad) seizure but is now called a *major motor seizure*. A typical major motor seizure involves almost the entire brain (*generalized seizure*), but sometimes it starts in one area of the brain (*focal seizure*) and then spreads to other areas or to the entire cortex (*focal seizure with secondary generalization*). If a seizure starts in one area of the brain, before the seizure becomes generalized, patients will sometimes have an *aura*. Depending on where the seizure focus is located in the brain, they may smell something strange, like a tire burning, or they may find that even familiar people and places look strange (*jamas vu*). When I asked Portia if she knew when she was going to have a seizure, she said, "Yes. The first thing I notice is a terrible feeling of fear. This lasts for a few seconds, and then I go out." Having a seizure is usually a very unpleasant event with negative social implications. The term *seizure* is an ancient one, deriving from the belief that the person with this condition has been seized by the devil. Although most people now recognize that this is not true, there is still a bias against

people with epilepsy. I asked Portia if she became frightened because she knew she was going to have a seizure. She said, "No. The
first warning I get is the feeling of intense fear. That's when I know
that I will probably have a seizure. The fear comes first, the concern
about a seizure second." This experience is not unique to Portia.
Many patients who have focal seizures, with or without secondary
generalization, have a feeling of fear before the convulsions begin.

We tried to control Portia's seizure with antiepileptic drugs. A
combination of hydantoin (Dilantin) and phenobarbital seemed to
work best. These drugs prevented some of the focal seizures from
becoming generalized motor seizures, but they did little to stop the
focal seizures. Because Portia's seizures were frequent and disabling,
we considered surgery. For more than 50 years, neurosurgeons have
been treating patients with focal seizures uncontrolled with drugs
by removing the part of the brain where the seizure starts. A seizure
that starts with the feeling of fear often originates from the anterior
part of the temporal lobe in a structure called the *amygdala* (Fig. 3–
2). Like other seizures, it can be traced and localized with an EEG.
Portia's EEG indicated that her seizures were starting in the right
anterior temporal lobe, but occasionally she also had abnormal EEG
activity in the left anterior temporal lobe. Because the surgeons did
not want to remove the area of Portia's brain that was not causing
the seizure, they placed several electrodes into the amygdala and
found that the seizures were originating from the amygdala on the

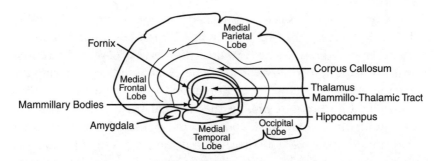

Figure 3–2. Diagram of the amygdala nucleus, which is located in the middle front part of the temporal lobe. In this diagram the brain is cut in half
(from front to back) along the long axis (sagittal section). The diagram demonstrates what the hemisphere looks like from the middle. When a seizure starts
in this nucleus, the first symptom the person may experience is a feeling of
overwhelming fear.

right side. The surgeons also stimulated part of the amygdala by delivering a small electrical current through a needle they had inserted into it. This amygdala stimulation caused Portia to feel fear. After they removed the amygdala in the right hemisphere, Portia was free of seizures. She graduated from Northeastern and is able to lead a normal life.

The amygdala, located below the cerebral cortex in the temporal lobe, is important in controlling visceral activation. It also feeds information about the viscera back to the cortex. The first symptom of patients like Portia is an emotional experience. This observation is inconsistent with Schacter's attribution-feedback theory because these patients felt an emotion in the absense of a stimulus or event to account for the increased visceral arousal. According to Schacter's theory, these patients should have had "as if" experiences. Feeling an emotion at the beginning of a seizure suggests that the attribution-feedback theory cannot entirely account for emotional experience, but it is still possible that feedback and attribution may modify or enrich emotional experiences.

Central Nervous System Theories

Although the amygdala is important in experiencing fear, the cerebral cortex must also be involved because emotions are conscious experiences. Much has been learned about the role of the cerebral cortex in the experience of emotion from observing patients with brain damage.

Cortical injury is often associated with sadness and depression. This was the case with Colonel Thomas Whitehouse, a patient at the Gainesville Veterans Affairs Medical Center. A 72-year-old retired Army officer, he had served with General George Patton during the Second World War, fought in Korea, and even spent time in Vietnam. His wife brought him to the hospital because his right arm had suddenly become weak and he could not speak. The symptoms had started about 24 hours earlier, but she had trouble persuading him to come to the hospital. When I first saw Colonel Whitehouse, he was sobbing and looked very frightened. I asked him if he was worried about his weakness and speech problem. He nodded. To make certain that he understood me, I gave him a few simple commands such as "Point to the door" and "Point to the ceiling." He performed all these simple tasks very well, but when I gave him more complex commands with multiple parts or complicated grammar, he had trouble understanding me. To see how well he could speak, I asked him to tell me what he had done during the Second World War. He said, "fight . . . Europe . . . Patton." I asked if he went to Germany. He said, "Yes . . . Germany." Then he started crying again and said, "Shit." I asked if talking about the war usually made him sad. He said, "No . . . like . . . war stories." Then why was he so sad? I asked. He pointed to his mouth. I said, "Because you are having trouble speaking." He nodded and said, "Yes." Then he pointed to his weak right arm and I said, "Because your arm is also weak." He nodded again.

The colonel's sudden loss of speech fluency together with his right arm weakness indicated that he had suffered damage from a stroke to Broca's area, which is instrumental in programming speech, as well as to the part of the motor cortex that controls the arm. Both of the damaged brain structures are on the lower left side of the frontal lobe. Later that day, a CT scan confirmed the diagnosis and the localization of the damage.

When I examined the colonel, I noted that he had some reflexes in his right hand and some movement of his fingers. I told him that these were good signs and that he would probably recover the use of his right arm. I also told him that we would start speech therapy and that the brain damage was so small that there was a good chance of recovering most of his speech. He started crying again and said, "Thank you. Thank you . . . try . . . make feel better." Even with this good news, however, he still seemed depressed. I asked his wife if he had had episodes of depression before the strokes. She answered, "No, he is one of the most stable and stoic men you will ever meet."

Several neurologists have noted that people with aphasia from left hemisphere lesions often become depressed and the depression is most likely to accompany damage to the frontal lobe. That was where the colonel had sustained damage. When patients work on their deficits they usually feel better, so I asked our speech pathologists, physical therapists, and occupational therapists to start working with the colonel as soon as possible. Nonetheless, he remained depressed, agitated, and anxious. He had no appetite and hardly ate. To alleviate his sadness and help his condition, I treated him with an antidepressant, which helped him to sleep, increased his appetite, and after about a week or two started to relieve his depression.

In contrast to a left hemisphere stroke, which induces depression, injury to the right hemisphere causes emotional indifference or even euphoria. Twenty years ago, the Shands Teaching Hospital received a call from a clinic on Nassau, one of the Carribean islands, stating that they were sending us a young Jesuit priest who had incurred brain or spinal cord damage from a scuba diving mishap. While scuba diving, he had come to the surface too quickly and developed a decompression illness. The physician on the island said that he was weak on his left side and had neck pain. He was sent to Shands because it was the hospital closest to the island that had a hyperbaric chamber. The priest was transported to Gainesville in a plane that was pressurized and flew low. On arrival, the emergency room staff rushed him to the hyperbaric chamber. While he was being treated with hyperbaric oxygen, the nurse noticed that his pupils were asymmetrical, the left larger than the right. This prompted a request for a neurological consultation.

The priest was 29 years old. Born in Ireland, he had spent part of his childhood in England but attended Georgetown University in Washington, D.C. He had been in the West Indies attempting to develop a liberal arts graduate program in one of the islands' universities. He liked the Carribean because he enjoyed diving. After introducing myself I asked, "When did you first notice any problems?" He replied, "I was fine until I started to come up. The first thing I noticed was pain on the right side my neck. A few minutes after that I noticed that, my left arm went numb and weak." I asked how deep the dive was and how long he had been underwater at that depth. "I don't think I went much past 50 feet and was down for no more than 20 minutes. I was coming up to the boat to get more film for my underwater camera." I asked if he had used decompression tables. "At that depth and with only one tank, I thought it would be hard to get into trouble. Instead of tables, I followed the old rule of staying behind the smallest bubble." He paused and then said, "but I guess I was wrong."

When I examined his eyes, I saw that the nurse was correct. The left pupil was larger that the right. Small asymmetries of pupil size (e.g., 1 mm) are commonly seen and may be normal, but in this patient the difference was large, about 3 to 4 mm. The left pupil can be larger than the right pupil either because the nerves that constrict the left pupil are injured or because the nerves that dilate the right pupil are not working properly. The nerve that moves the eye toward the nose also carries the nerve fibers that constrict the pupil. If the patient's left pupil was abnormally enlarged because this nerve had been damaged, he should have been unable to move this eye toward his nose. To learn if this nerve had been injured, I asked him to watch my finger while I moved it in different directions. Since he could move his left eye toward his nose, this nerve was apparently normal. The nerve that dilates the pupil does not travel to the eye with any of the nerves that move the eye; therefore, it was probably the small pupil in the right eye that was abnormal. The nerve that dilates the pupil goes to the right eye by traveling along the *carotid artery*, the major artery that supplies blood to the cerebral hemisphere. Sometimes in young people, for unknown reasons, the carotid artery tears and then a clot may form within it. This tear is called a *carotid dissection*. Such tearing is often associated with neck pain similar to the one this young priest had experienced. Because the neck pain was on the same side as the small pupil, and because he was weak on the opposite side, I thought that he had had a right carotid dissection. In order to make this diagnosis, the radiologist injected dye into this vessel and took x-rays of his neck and head (arteriography). The team of physicians and nurses who staffed the hyperbaric chamber were at first reluctant to order this procedure because they thought the patient might benefit from another course of hyperbaric treatment. However, I stated that he did not have the symptoms of the bends and that if he had a carotid dissection, it would have to be treated with anticoagulants so that the entire artery did not close or send a big clot up to his brain. They agreed to transfer him to the neurology service and an emergency angiographic study was performed. It showed that the carotid artery was torn. A CT scan of his brain revealed that a small stroke had injured the lower part of the motor cortex. This stroke was probably caused by a clot that had broken off from the torn artery. Unfortunately, shortly after this study and before an anticoagulant could be given, he suffered a second, larger stroke that increased his weakness.

For a few days after the second stroke the priest was somewhat lethargic, but then he became more alert. I spoke to him about his weakness, but he appeared to be totally unconcerned about the stroke and at times appeared to think that it was funny. Sometimes patients with right hemisphere strokes are unaware of their disabilities, but the priest knew that he had had a stroke. He was an exceptionally intelligent man with a wealth of information, and I was curious to learn if his indifference and inappropriate jocularity were limited to his illness. Our conversations ranged over many topics, each of which he discussed in an enlightened manner, but I never saw any signs of concern, sadness, or anger even when we talked about issues that ordinarily evoke such responses. For example, he had a sister with leukemia but expressed no sadness when talking about her or her disease. I asked why he did not seem sad when he spoke about his sister, who was so close to him. His answer was that he knew Jesus would take care of her. I asked if he missed her and he said, "No, not now."

The priest's parents lived in Ireland. When they heard that he had suffered a stroke, they came here to visit him. Both his mother and father were warm, caring people. After discussing his medical condition with them, I took them to his room for a visit. The following day, after examining the priest to make certain that he had not developed any new neurological symptoms and had no evidence of abnormal bleeding, we told him and his family that he was stable and that there appeared to be no new complications from the treatment. When we left the room, his parents asked to speak with me, and we met a few hours later after I finished rounds. His father said, "He looks like our son and has the same voice as our son, but he is not the same person we knew and loved." Continuing, he said, "He's not the same person he was before he had this stroke. Our son was a warm, caring, and sensitive person. All that is gone. He now sounds like a robot." I explained that the right hemisphere is important in expressing facial emotions and generating emotional prosody in speech. "Yes, I know," he replied. "Your resident told us that he had these emotional expressive problems, but it is more than that. When we spoke about his duties as a priest and said he may not be able to perform his duties, he said, 'So what?' He has a younger sister who has leukemia. He is crazy about her, or maybe I should say, was. She was in remission when he came to the West Indies, but now she is also in the hospital with a relapse. At first, we were hesitant to tell him because we didn't want to upset him, but I was surprised that he never asked about her, so I decided to tell him. He never asked how she was doing, and the only thing he said after we told him about her condition was, 'Is Jim Thomas still taking care of her? What a character Jim is. Always had the best jokes. Do you want to hear one?' I told him, no! I was in no mood for jokes. He said,

'Shame.' That's not the way our son acted before he became sick."
I told the couple that some people with right hemisphere injury like
their son, lose their emotions and appear either inappropriately flat
or inappropriately euphoric and jocular. Weeping, the mother
asked, "Will he get better?" My answer was, "I hope so." The mother
left Gainesville early so that she could be with her daughter, who
died a few months later. When the priest was discharged the following week his father took him back to Ireland. I never learned the
outcome of his case.

The colonel and the priest illustrate a phenomenon that has
been repeatedly reported: patients with left hemisphere damage are
often sad and anxious, while those with right hemisphere damage
can be either calm-indifferent or inappropriately happy. D. Frank
Benson, as well as Sergio Starkstein and his colleagues, have reported that the areas of the brain where injuries induce these emotions are located in the frontal lobes. Based on these clinical observations, investigators have suggested that the left hemisphere
normally mediates positive emotions (e.g., happiness, joy), while the
right hemisphere mediates negative ones (e.g., fear, anger, sadness).
Injury to one hemisphere disinhibits, or releases from control, the
other hemisphere. Using electrophysiological techniques in normal
subjects, Richard Davidson has shown that positive emotions are associated with left frontal lobe activation and negative emotions with
right frontal lobe activation. When an area of the brain becomes
active, blood flow to that area increases. Positron emission tomography has been used to study emotion. With this technology John
Mazziotta found that in people experiencing sadness and depression, blood flow to the left frontal lobe was decreased, suggesting
that this part of the brain was not being normally activated.

Most of us are capable of experiencing several different negative and positive emotions. The negative ones include sadness, anger, disgust, and fear; the positive ones include contentment, happiness, joy, and pleasant surprise. The frontal lobe valence theory
cannot explain how we feel all these different emotions. When we
experience some emotions, such as fear or surprise, we are excited
and alert. When we experience other emotions, such as sadness and
boredom, we are more lethargic. About 100 years ago, Hans Berger
noticed that small amounts of electricity could be detected by placing electrodes on the scalp and amplifying the small currents these
electrodes recorded from the brain. The amount of current detected

and recorded by this amplifier changed several times per second and resembled a series of waves on a graph. These recordings are called *electroencephalograms* (EEGs). Investigators noticed that when the subject became drowsy, the waves occurred about four to eight times, or cycles, per second. If the subject was awake but relaxed, the EEG waves cycled at a rate of about 8 to 12 times per second, but if he or she was excited, the wave cycle was more rapid and less well defined. About 50 years ago, Moruzzi and Magoun placed electrodes in the *midbrain reticular formation* of a cat (Fig. 3–3). The midbrain is located immediately below the cerebral hemispheres. When electric current was sent into the electrodes, the drowsy cat became awake and excited. Electrophysiologists recording electrical impulses from the cortex using the EEG found that when an animal is alert, the nerve cells in the cortex are more excitable; that is, they are more prepared to discharge, or fire, and carry impulses from neuron to neuron. All sensory systems send signals to the midbrain reticular formation. Thus, an external stimulus can excite the reticular formation and arouse the cortex. The nerves cells in the cortex, however, also send projections (axons) to the reticular formation, allowing thoughts to activate this structure.

When people becomes excited, their palms sweat. We can measure this sweat by placing by two electrodes on the hand and measure how efficiently the skin conducts small amounts of electricity. The more someone sweats, the better the conductance. This mea-

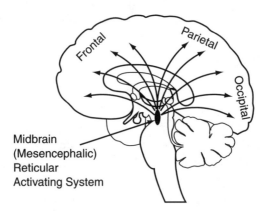

Midbrain
(Mesencephalic)
Reticular
Activating System

Figure 3–3. Diagram of a sagittal section of the brain in which the brain is cut in half (from front to back) along the long axis, showing the reticular activating system in the midbrain. This reticular system is responsible for arousing the cerebral cortex.

surement is called the *electrodermal response* or *galvanic skin response* (GSR). The GSR correlates very well with central measures of arousal such as the EEG. When the GSR is high the EEG waves are fast, a sign of arousal, and when the GSR is low the EEG waves are slow. To learn which areas of the cortex have the most control over arousal or excitement, we gave people with strokes in different brain regions a mild electric shock to their normal hand. The strength of the shock was determined by each patient so that the shock was uncomfortable but not painful. We found that patients with strokes of the right hemisphere had much smaller GSR responses to the shock than those with left hemisphere strokes or normal controls. In addition, patients with left hemisphere strokes had greater GSR responses than controls. These results suggest that while the right hemisphere controls the reticular activating system, the left hemisphere inhibits the right hemisphere. Thus, when highly arousing emotions (e.g., fear) are experienced, the right hemisphere is activated, and when emotions with low arousal (e.g., contentment) are experienced, the activated left hemisphere inhibits the right hemisphere and the reticular formation is downregulated.

Although many emotions may be defined by valence (positive and negative) and by the degree of arousal (high and low), these two factors alone cannot fully explain the wide range of emotional experiences. For example, anger and fear are both negative in valence and associated with high arousal, but they are associated with different experiences or feelings. Thus, other elements must also be important in the experience of emotion.

I learned about a third element that might be important in the experience of emotion when, as a visiting professor at a northeastern medical school and hospital, I examined a 22-year-old woman named Mary Jackson. Having grown up in a poor inner-city neighborhood, she was the valedictorian of her high school class and a leader in student government. She had received a scholarship to an Ivy League university. In her first 2 years there she did extremely well and was on the dean's list in all four semesters. Although her major was history, she was also taking premedical courses because she wanted to go to medical school, become a pediatrician, and work with inner-city children. Her boyfriend, Tom, was attending another university in the same metropolitan area, and they planned to marry after she completed medical school. In the summer between her sophomore and junior years, Tom and another friend began to see some changes in her behavior. She started to go to bars, first on weekends and then during the week. She also began to pick up men at these bars, often ending up in bed with them. She and her family were Baptists and she had rarely drank alcohol, but now she started drinking regularly in large amounts. Her family was unaware of these behavioral changes, but Tom became increasingly concerned. He thought that she had rejected him, and they broke up. Her behavior, however, continued to deteriorate.

One day when Tom dropped in to see how she was doing, he spotted some powder in a tube that looked like cocaine. Mary admitted that it was but said she was holding it for a friend. Tom pleaded with her to get professional help, but she ordered him to leave and never return. In her next semester in college, she got an F in three courses and a D in two. Her advisor warned her that if her grades did not improve, she would lose her scholarship. He also recommended counseling, but she refused and became verbally abusive.

In the second semester of her junior year, Mary slept through almost all her classes. One day she developed a high fever, chills, and a cough. The physician at the student health service asked whether she had noticed any problems earlier. Mary said that she had been tired but simply had been partying too much. She also told him that she had not had a menstrual period (*amenorrhea*) for 4 or 5 months. The doctor examined her and ordered an x-ray of her lungs and blood tests. After reviewing the results, the physician diagnosed pneumonia and admitted her to the hospital. He said that she needed to be treated with an intravenous antibiotic and oxygen. He also wanted to find out why she had gotten pneumonia and was not menstruating.

In the hospital, Mary was given oxygen through a nasal cannula and intravenous fluids with an antibiotic. Additional blood and urine tests were performed. Mary's type of pneumonia is often associated with acquired immune deficiency syndrome (AIDS), and in young women the most common reason for failure to menstruate is pregnancy. Mary was not pregnant, but unfortunately her human immunodeficiency virus (HIV) test was positive. The physician asked Mary if she used drugs. She admitted to snorting cocaine but denied ever injecting it or sharing a needle. The doctor asked if she had slept with men to make money to support her drug habit. She admitted sleeping around but not for money. She cried and said that she did not understand why she was promiscuous. This had never happened when she was younger, but now she could no longer turn down the men she met in bars. Was the AIDS causing her amenorrhea? The doctor was not sure of the reason, but hoped that the results of some of the hormone tests would be helpful. She asked to see a psychiatrist, and the physician thought this was an excellent idea.

The psychiatrist who came to see Mary spoke with her for about 30 minutes. After this interview, he wrote a note in her chart that reviewed her history, diagnosed her as having a "borderline personality disorder," and recommended outpatient psychotherapy.

The next morning, Mary's physician reported that her amenorrhea might be due to a problem with her pituitary, or master gland. He had asked a neurologist to see her and had ordered an MRI scan of her brain.

Pituitary tumors can cause constriction of the visual fields. If I asked you to look straight ahead, put your hands behind your ears, and then slowly bring them forward, you would normally start seeing your hands when they were 3 or 4 inches in front of your ears. When Mary did this, she could not see my hands until they were almost in front of her eyes. Also, when I touched her palm with my index and middle fingers, she closed her hand around my fingers—the grasp reflex. When I hit her ankle (Achilles) tendon with my reflex hammer her reflexes were slow.

I gave Mary some mental status tests. She was oriented and knew the date and place. I gave her three objects to remember (daisy, lamp, and mirror) and then distracted her by asking her to count backward from 100 by sevens. When I asked her to recall the three objects, she could only recall one. When I wanted to test her memory again, she got very angry and said, "Once is enough." After I explained the importance of this test she agreed, but her performance was the same. I asked if she noticed that her memory was getting bad, and she said "No." Seeing how easily she was provoked to anger, I asked if she had a "short fuse." She said, "Up to about a year ago, it was extremely rare that I got angry. Now it seems I am always flying off the handle." Because she had a grasp reflex, a sign of frontal lobe dysfunction, I also performed some tests of frontal lobe function. François Lhermitte, a Parisian neurologist, noted that patients with frontal lobe injuries tended to approach and use objects abnormally. To test Mary for this abnormal approach and utilization behavior, I put some objects on a table in front of her but said nothing about using them. When I put a pen and paper on the table without giving any instructions, she picked up the pen and starting writing. When I asked the reason she said, "I thought you wanted to see me write." I replied, "No. If I want you to do something, I will ask you." A few minutes later, I put a comb on the table in front of her; she picked it up and started combing her hair. It seemed that rather than having internal goals motivate her behavior, she was stimulus dependent—often a sign of frontal lobe dysfunction. Lhermitte called this abnormal behavior the *environmental dependancy syndrome*. To further test Mary's stimulus dependence, I told her to make a fist. Then I asked her to raise one finger as soon as I held up two fingers and to raise two fingers when I held up one. She often mimicked my movements but then corrected her performance. I also gave her the Stroop test, in which color names (i.e., red, blue, and green) are printed in a color that is different from their meaning. For example, the word *red* might be printed in blue and the word *green* in red. I asked Mary to go down the list of these words but, rather than reading the words, to name the colors in which the words were printed. She performed very poorly on this test, often reading the word rather than naming the color.

Mary's personality changes included a reduction of frustration tolerance with an increased propensity to anger, a decline in long-term goal-oriented behaviors, and an inability to avoid seductive situations. These changes are often associated with injury to the ventral areas of the frontal lobes. Because these area are directly over the eye orbits, they are called *orbitofrontal cortices*.

After patients are infected with HIV, the virus can travel to and infect the brain. The first signs of brain infection that many patients with HIV-AIDS demonstrate are symptoms of frontal lobe and memory dysfunction—Mary's symptoms. Although it was possible that Mary had the beginning of an AIDS dementia, this diagnosis could not explain her abnormal vision. The loss of lateral vision is often caused by pressure on the optic nerves. Tumors of the pituitary can press on the optic nerves, and if they are large enough they can also press on the orbitofrontal cortex. Since the pituitary is the master gland, a tumor could also explain why Mary was no longer menstruating and why her reflexes were slow, a sign that the thyroid gland was not working properly.

An MRI scan revealed that Mary had an extremely large tumor that appeared to be orignate from the pituitary (Fig. 3–4). It was

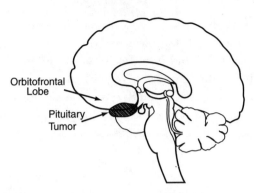

Orbitofrontal
Lobe

Pituitary
Tumor

Figure 3–4. Diagram of Mary's brain. The brain is cut in half (from front to back) along the long axis. The diagram shows the tumor pressing on the orbitofrontal cortex.

pressing on the optic nerves and the orbitofrontal cortex. This tumor could account for almost all of Mary's symptoms, including what the psychiatrist had diagnosed as borderline personality disorder.

After returning to Gainesville, I inquired about Mary. She underwent neurosurgery to remove the tumor, began hormone replacement therapy, and was given antiviral treatment for her HIV infection. She has been doing very well. She went back to college, got her degree, and is now working on a master's degree in social work. Her mother thinks that she still loses her temper more rapidly than she did before the tumor developed, but in general says her daughter is "her old self."

I think Derek Denny-Brown had provided the best explanation of why frontal lobe injury causes the abnormal behavior displayed by Mary. When confronted with a stimulus, almost all animals, including humans, have a propensity to either approach or avoid it. Denny-Brown suggested that whereas the frontal lobes mediate avoidance behavior, the parietal lobes mediate approach behavior. When the frontal lobes are injured, especially the orbitofrontal cortex, inappropriate approach behavior develops, as displayed by Mary both in the physical examination (grasp reflex) and during mental status testing (utilization behavior). Her stimulus dependence and inability to achieve long-term goals might have accounted for many of her behavioral changes including school failure, promiscuity, and illicit drug use. In the emotional domain, approach-avoidance is par-

allel to fight or flight. When confronted with a stimulus that induces
a negative emotion with high arousal, one can either approach and
fight (anger) or avoid and flee (fear). Some of Mary's other behavioral problems might have been related to her aberrant approach
tendency. Situations that should have caused her fear were not
avoided. She was stimulus bound and, like many patients with orbitofrontal injuries, she often became inappropriately angry.

Summary

Much of human emotional experience can be explained by the
three factors that we have discussed: valence (pleasant versus unpleasant), arousal (high versus low), and action (approach versus
avoidance). Valence is mediated by the dorsolateral frontal lobes.
Activation of the left frontal lobe induces positive feelings, and activation of the right frontal lobe creates negative feelings. The as-
cending reticular formation, located in the midbrain, modulates cortical arousal. The right hemisphere is important for activating the
reticular formation, and the left hemisphere inhibits the right hemisphere. Avoidance behaviors are controlled by the frontal lobes, especially the orbitofrontal cortex, and the parietal cortex programs
approach behaviors. Although we have focused on the anatomical
areas comprising the modular systems that mediate these three factors, studies of patients with mood disorders have shown that ma-
nipulation of neurotransmitters (chemicals that send messages from
one nerve to another nerve) such as serotonin may strongly influence the experience of emotion. The mechanisms by which these
neurotransmitters influence mood, however, remain unclear.

Selected Readings

Borod, J. (2000) *The neuropsychology of emotions,* Oxford University
    Press, New York.
Bowers, D., Bauer, R.M., Heilman, K.M. (1993) The non-verbal af-
    fect lexicon: Theoretical perspectives from neuropsychological
    studies of affect perception. *Neuropsychology* 7:433–444.
Heilman, K.M., Bowers, D., Valenstein, E. (1993) Emotional disor-
    ders associated with neurological diseases. In *Clinical Neuropsy-
    chology.* (Ed.) Heilman, K.M., and Valenstein, E., Oxford Univer-
    sity Press, New York, pp. 461–497.
LeDoux, J.E. (1996) *The emotional brain,* Simon & Shuster, New York.

CHAPTER
4

ATTENTION

William James, a Harvard-trained physician and one of the founders of American psychology, said that *attention* is one of those terms that is difficult to define, though everybody knows what it means. This term may be difficult to define because, rather than being an object, it is a process that is not well understood. Humans need to use attentional processing because our brains have a limited capacity. That is, they receive more information than they can process simultaneously and fully. While you are reading this book, if you find it interesting, you are attending to the words on the page and are unaware of how your left foot feels—until I mention your left foot. Now you can shift your attention to it and feel it. In this chapter we will discuss how we become aware of stimuli, focus our attention, and withdraw it.

SENSORY AWARENESS

Clinical Observations of Unawareness

When I was a medical student at the University of Virginia, there was a hierarchy, and the medical students were at the bottom. To make it easier for the house staff and faculty to recognize us, we wore short white coats with normally colored pants such as chinos. The interns, residents, and fellows wore short white coats with white pants. It was easy, however, to tell the interns from the residents and fellows. They always looked tired, and their whites never seemed to be as white as the residents' uniforms. The attending physicians, who were the faculty of the medical school, wore long, white, neatly pressed coats. The dress code allowed the medical staff and patients to know that we were students.

On the way to picking up a bottle of urine from a patient, I passed a middle-aged man who was sitting on the edge of his bed eating his lunch. He said, "Doc, can you come over here?" I looked around to see if any of the house staff or attending physicians were nearby, but I was the only one on the ward at that time, so I walked over to the man's bed and said, "I am not a doctor yet, but I would be happy to try and help you." He said, "Being a medical student is good enough for me to call you 'Doc.' " When I thanked him and offered to help, he asked, "What kind of weird place is this? Look at my food tray. They only served me vegetables. I am not on a special diet. How do I get some meat?" I looked down at his tray. On it was a hospital plate with a divider to separate the ground-up meat from the ground-up vegetables. The vegetables were on the right side of the plate and the meat, which didn't look quite edible, was on the left side. On rounds, I had heard that this man had been admitted after a stroke. I thought that perhaps the stroke had injured the right occipital lobe, containing the visual cortex, which is important for seeing the left side. Because I thought that the patient could not see on the left side, I rotated the dish 180 degrees so that meat was now on the right side. He said, "Thank you, Doctor, for finding me some meat."

When this man finished eating, I came back to examine him. Blindness on one side is called *hemianopia* (loss of half vision). This loss of vision usually occurs in both eyes. To test the patient for hemianopia, I stood facing him and asked him to look at my nose.

I then told him that I would move either my right or my left hand, and he was to tell me which hand I moved. When I moved my right hand, which normal people see with their right occipital cortex, he had no problem seeing my moving hand. Since his left-sided vision was normal, I did not understand why he could not see the left side of his plate. The other main finding of my examination was severe weakness of the patient's left arm, which he kept in a flexed posture on his chest.

The attending physician that month was a New Zealander named Dr. Fritz Dreyfus, a superb neurologist and teacher. The next day, at the end of rounds, when he asked if anyone had questions, I asked him to explain why this patient, who was not blind on his left side, could not see the meat on the left side of his plate. Even when physicians cannot explain symptoms, they can name them. For example, some people might develop red bumps on their skin. The dermatologist who examines them may not know what is causing the rash but will tell them that they have erythema nodosum, which in Latin means red bumps. Dr. Dreyfus said that the man had what is called *unilateral neglect.* He added that Derek Denny-Brown, the most famous neurologist from New Zealand, had written about this disorder, and he suggested that I read his articles.

After we finished rounds, I went to the library and started reading everything I could find about unilateral neglect. I learned that when patients with this condition try to draw or copy a figure, they often leave out the side of the picture opposite the side of their brain injury (contralesional). In another test for unilateral neglect, patients are shown a horizontal line and asked to locate its center. The patients with neglect respond by deviating their mark to the non-neglected side of the line, an ipsilateral spatial bias. Lastly, there is the cancellation test, developed by Simon Horenstein and later reported by Martin Albert to be a sensitive indicator of neglect. In this test, the physician draws many small lines, about 1 or 2 inches long, and distributes them randomly over a page of white paper. He or she then shows the patients this paper and asks them to cross out, or cancel, all of the lines. Patients with neglect fail to cross out the lines on the side of the page opposite to their brain lesion.

I went back to the wards to see the man with unilateral neglect. After speaking with him for several minutes about the reasons he came to the hospital, I was surprised that he appeared so calm and indifferent when his left side was so weak. His name was George Jones, and he was a 67-year-old retired civil engineer. I asked him if I could perform some tests and he replied, "Yes, you are the doctor." I also received approval from the medical team that was taking care of him.

The first test I gave him was the line bisection test. I drew a line about 10 inches long on a blank piece of paper, put it in front of him, gave him a pencil, and asked him to put a mark in the middle of the line. He said, "Doc, you mean bisect the line." I nodded. He said, "Doc, you probably remember from geometry that the way you bisect a line is to draw either an equilateral or isosceles triangle and then drop a meridian." He then proceeded to draw an isosceles triangle. The two sides of the triangle were equal, as they should be. But whereas the right leg of the triangle did come down to the right end of the horizontal line, the left leg of the triangle came down to the middle of the line rather than to the left end. Therefore, when the patient dropped his meridian, it intersected the horizontal line several inches to the right of center. He then darkened this intersection of the horizontal line and his meridian, pointed to this intersection with the index finger of his right hand, and said, "There, the line has been bisected" (Fig. 4–1). Considering how he missed seeing the meat on the left side of the plate, his performance on this line bisection task was not surprising. Mr. Jones's performance illustrates that if you initially misperceive the world, even if you perform formal operations your behavior remains deviant.

Next, I drew a simple picture of a daisy and asked him to copy

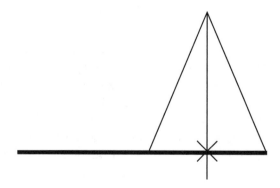

Figure 4–1. A reproduction of Mr. Jones's attempt to bisect the line by first drawing an isosceles triangle and then dropping a meridian. However, because the left end of the triangle was not on the left end of the line, his meridian is not at the midpoint of the line.

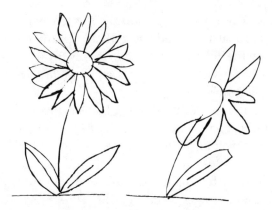

Figure 4–2. A reproduction of Mr. Jones's attempt to copy the picture of the daisy that I had drawn.

it. His drawing showed neglect (see Fig. 4–2). He did not draw petals on the left side of the flower, and he placed the drawing on the far right side of the page. Lastly, I gave Mr. Jones the cancellation test; he canceled only the lines on the right side of the page (Fig. 4–3).

Brain Mechanisms

It was apparent that Mr. Jones was unaware of stimuli on the left side. But why? That weekend, admissions to the hospital slowed down and I was able to read more about this unilateral, or hemi-spatial, neglect. Denny-Brown wrote that after somatosensory (touch, pain, heat/cold, position), visual, and auditory stimuli come to the cerebral cortex, this sensory information converges in the

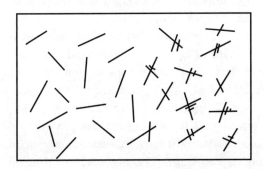

Figure 4–3. A reproduction of a cancellation test. Mr. Jones was asked to cancel all the lines. He failed to cancel the lines on the left side of the page.

parietal lobes. The senses that monitor the left half of space meet in the right parietal lobe, and those that monitor the right half of space meet in the left parietal lobe. Denny-Brown suggested that this multimodal sensory synthesis allows us to develop awareness of the right and left halves of space.

While I was in medical school, I had no further opportunities to learn about neglect. After training in internal medicine, I decided to become a neurologist. I took my residency at the Harvard Neurological Unit of Boston City Hospital because that was where Denny-Brown was Chairman. During my residency, I was asked to see a patient on the medical service. The patient was brought to the hospital by his family because he had sudden onset of left-sided weakness, or hemiplegia. After performing a physical examination, I tested this patient using some of the same tests I had used with Mr. Jones. On the line bisection task, he thought that the midline was 2 inches to the right of the actual midline. On the line cancellation test, he canceled only the lines on the right half of the page. Like Mr. Jones, he was unaware of stimuli on the left side of space. When I asked why he came to the hospital, he replied, "Because my family brought me." I diagnosed this patient as having had a stroke of the right parietal lobe. Shortly after completing my evaluation and writing a note on his chart, I received a call from the medical resident caring for this patient. He asked if I wanted to obtain a radioisotope scan of his brain. Compared to today's brain imaging methods this radioisotope scanning was not very revealing, and I felt confident that the patient had had a stroke that injured his right parietal lobe. In addition, radioisotope scanning was not available in Boston City Hospital. Therefore, I, told the medical resident that I was pretty confident about my diagnosis and did not think there was any need for a radioisotope scan.

Two days later, I again saw this medical resident, who was carrying an x-ray film. He caught up with me and said, "Ken, remember my patient with left-sided neglect whom you saw a couple of days ago?" I nodded. He said, "Well guess what?" This question was cause for panic. Before CT imaging was available, neurologists were frequently concerned that by relying on the physical history and examination alone, they might have missed a tumor or blood clot that could be removed surgically. The main way to find out if a patient had such a lesion was to perform a test called an *angiogram* or *arteriogram*. It involved injecting a dye directly into the carotid artery in the neck, which carries blood to the brain, and then obtaining a series of x-rays of the skull. The dye allowed us to see the arteries. In addition to seeing if an artery was blocked, we could see if the arteries were being displaced by a tumor or blood clot. Although the arteriogram was a good diagnostic test, about 3%–5% of the patients who were given it in our hospital had a serious side effect such as a stroke. Thus, we did not use this test if we thought the patient had already had a stroke, but only when we believed there was a strong possibility of a tumor or a blood clot on the surface of the brain. I asked the resident if he had the results of an arteriogram on the x-rays. He said, "No, not an arteriogram; it is a radioisotope scan." He then gave it to me. Rather than showing a stroke that had damaged the parietal lobe, the scan revealed damage to the frontal lobe. I said, "I never knew that patients could get neglect from damage to their frontal lobe. I need to review the literature to see what I can find. Can you get me a copy of this scan?" The resident said, "This is your copy. I thought you would want one." I said, "Thanks! How did you get this scan?" He answered, "Don't ask."

The next weekend, I was on call. This meant staying and sleeping in the hospital for more than 48 hours. All the patients on our inpatient service were stable. There were only a few consultations and calls from the emergency room, so I could spend a lot of time in the library. One of the modern inventions for which I am most thankful is the Medline service. If you want to review all the articles written on neglect, all you have to do is log on to Medline and type the words *neglect* and *frontal lobe*. The computer will search the National Library of Medicine, and within seconds will display all the articles written on this subject since the 1960s. Although the full articles are not always available, you can get an abstract. If the abstract looks interesting, you can read the journal in the library. In the 1960s, however, it was necessary to search through a set of thick, heavy books called *Index Medicus*. Each year a new volume appeared. I had to go through ten of these books but found nothing about the frontal lobes and neglect. In general, there was also very little about neglect alone.

By the time I had seen this man with frontal lobe neglect, Denny-Brown had retired as Chairman of Boston City Hospital's Harvard Neurological Unit and Norman Geschwind, who had been Chairman at Boston University, had taken over his position. One of the nice customs Dr. Geschwind started was to have morning coffee in a small meeting room with several chairs around a table. During these times, a resident or faculty member could sit down and chat with him about anything that was on his or her mind. The day after seeing the scan on this man with the frontal stroke I attended this morning coffee. A good observer, Dr. Geschwind asked, "What's on your mind, Ken?" I told him about the patient with neglect having a frontal lesion and showed him the brain scan. He said, "Interesting. In almost all the reports of experimental neglect in monkeys, the neglect was induced by making frontal lobe lesions." Not wanting to spend another day with *Index Medicus* I asked, "Do you recall the reference?" He said, "Welch and Stuteville wrote a paper published in *Brain* about 10 to 15 years ago". Our departmental library had many older issues of *Brain*, and I had no difficulty finding the article. I made one copy for the medical resident and one copy for myself.

In most neurology journal articles, the author reviews the past literature before describing his or her new observations. Two things struck me about this article. Although previous investigators as far back as the late nineteenth century had reported neglect-like behavior in animals with frontal lesions, there was no mention that humans develop neglect if they have injuries in the same regions of the frontal lobes. In addition, the anatomical location of a posterior lesion that could induce neglect in monkeys was not entirely elucidated.

After Norman Geschwind came to Harvard, he recruited Deepak Pandya, a neuroanatomist who is interested in how different parts of the cerebral cortex are connected anatomically. Studying monkeys' brains, Pandya found that each of the primary sensory reception areas in the cerebral cortex areas projects only to its own association areas. Thus, the primary visual area is connected to visual association areas, the primary auditory area projects to the auditory association areas, and the primary somatosensory area (e.g., touch) projects to the somatosensory association areas (Fig. 4–4). Each of these sensory- or modality-specific association areas projects to multimodal (polymodal) or supramodal sensory areas. In humans, one of these polymodal sensory areas is located in the inferior portion of the parietal lobe (Fig. 4–4). Unlike the primary sensory reception areas, which perform analyses of stimuli, the modality specific sensory association areas perform syntheses, and these syntheses allow the brain to form percepts. The supramodal areas receive input about percepts from several modality-specific association areas, as

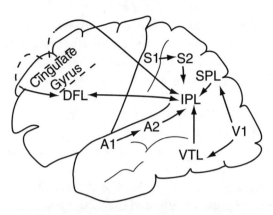

Figure 4-4. Diagram of cortical attention network. Visual, tactile, and auditory stimuli project to their primary sensory cortices, which are receiving areas that perform sensory analysis (visual primary cortex = V1, auditory = A1, tactile = S1). These primary cortical areas project to a higher level of cortex that helps synthesize sensory inputs and match them to stored memories, or representations, of previous experience in this modality (S2 = somatosensory association cortex, A2 = auditory association cortex, VTL + SPL = visual association cortex). Each of these sensory association areas then projects to a polymodal or supramodal area in the inferior parietal lobe (IPL), where sensory percepts activate higher concepts. This figure also demonstrates the strong connections between the frontal and parietal lobes (SPL = superior parietal lobe, VTL = ventral temporal lobe, DFL = dorsolateral frontal lobe).

well as input from other portions of the brain not directly related to sensory input. These supramodal areas allow people to make cross-modal associations (e.g., the shape of a dog and a bark) and help them determine the meaning of stimuli.

Primate brains are convoluted. A convoluted brain has mountains called *gyri*, valleys called *sulci*, and gorges called *fissures*. When I first visited my wife's family in West Virginia, I commented that West Virginia was a small state. My wife, who is proud of her home state, told me that if West Virginia was flattened, it might be larger than states without mountains such as Florida. That is, although West Virginia occupies a smaller space than Florida because it has so many mountains and valleys, its surface area is very large. The cerebral cortex of primates contains the neuronal systems that are critical for mediating complex activities. Therefore, as primate brains evolved, they needed more neuronal systems. An increase in neuronal systems allows greater intelligence by increasing the storage capacity of the brain and the ability to make computations. To increase the surface area, where the neurons are found, without greatly increasing the size of the head, the brain developed gyri, sulci, and fissures. The banks of the sulci are like the sides of the mountains.

Deepak Pandya demonstrated that in monkeys the polymodal areas, where all the senses come together, are located in the inferior parietal gyrus and in both banks of the superior temporal sulcus. The superior bank of the superior temporal sulcus is the superior temporal gyrus, and the inferior bank is the middle temporal gyrus. Reading Pandya's papers reminded me of the paper on neglect written by Denny-Brown, who suggested that all the sensory modalities come together in the parietal lobes of humans and that this synthesis allows us to be aware of stimuli in the opposite half of space. Since in monkeys all the senses come together in the banks of the superior temporal sulcus and the inferior parietal gyrus, if these regions are destroyed in one hemisphere (e.g., the right), the animal should neglect stimuli that are presented on the opposite (left) side of space.

To test this hypothesis, I asked Dr. Pandya if we could destroy this polymodal area, on one side of the brain, in a few rhesus monkeys and see if this injury induced neglect. In other (control) monkeys we could destroy an equal-sized area in a different part of the brain that is not polymodal. He agreed, and the experiments were performed. The monkeys that had the parietal-temporal lesions demonstrated unilateral neglect, and the control monkeys did not. These observations appeared to support Denny-Brown's hypothesis. When examined these monkeys, however, something troubled me. If a stimulus was presented to the side opposite their temporal-parietal lesions, the monkeys sometimes appeared to be aware of this stimulus. However, if both the right and left sides were stimulated at the same time, the animal only appeared to be aware of the stimulus on the same side of the body as the cerebral lesion (ipsilateral side). According to Denny-Brown's hypothesis, these temporal-parietal lesions should have destroyed the representation of contralateral space. If so, why could these monkeys sometimes detect a single stimulus applied to the side opposite the lesion, but, when given simultaneous stimuli on both sides, fail to detect the stimulus on the side opposite their hemispheric lesion? Denny-Brown's hypothesis could not entirely account for these observations.

This phenomenon of failing to sense a stimulus on one side when stimulated on both sides had been reported in humans by Morris Bender, a New York neurologist who practiced at Mount Sinai Hospital more than a half century ago. Dr. Bender called it *extinction to simultaneous stimulation* but did not speculate about the underlying mechanisms. However, Walther Poppelreuter an early-twentieth-century German neurologist, thought that unawareness of stimuli opposite a hemispheric lesion may be related to a defect in attention, but what *is* attention?

After finishing my internal medicine training and before beginning my neurology residency, I joined the Air Force. At this time, in the mid-1960s, I had to go to Alabama for basic training. Part of the training involved how to deal with a disaster when there are more injured people than can be cared for simultaneously with limited personal and supplies (limited capacity). In this situation, one doctor has to be the triage officer. As this officer examines the injured people, he or she categorizes them into four groups. *Minimal* means that the injuries are so minor that they will probably heal by themselves, without medical or surgical intervention. *Immediate* means that if the injured person does not get immediate attention, he or she will probably die or be permanently disabled. These are the people who must be treated first. *Expectant* means that the person is so badly injured that he or she will probably die despite intervention, or that caring for this person will be such a drain on the available resources that two or more people classified as immediate may die. *Delay* means that the person needs treatment but will still survive, with no or little disability, if treatment is delayed. Attention is, in part, a mental triage process. We attend to those external or internal stimuli that are most important to us. The significance of a stimulus is determined by several factors. We almost always attend to a novel stimulus because we have not yet determined its meaning. We also attend to stimuli that are important to us, as determined by our immediate needs (drives) and future goals.

When reading this book attending to your left foot is not important to you, so you are probably not aware of it, but if a bug crawled onto your foot you would immediately attend to your foot because you detected a new stimulus. If you had pain in this foot, you would attend to it because pain induces immediate needs or drives. If you were waiting for a salesperson to put on a new shoe, you would also attend to it because of future goals or motivations.

According to the Russian physiological psychologist Y.N. Soko-
lov, the sensory cortices and sensory association areas store memories of incoming stimuli. When a stimulus is new, the person develops an orienting response and attends to the stimulus. According to
our model, the information from sensory areas projects to the supramodal temporal-parietal region, which is critical in directing attention. In addition to receiving projections from the sensory association cortex, the temporal-parietal region receives strong
anatomical projections from the dorsolateral frontal lobe. The
temporal-parietal area also projects back to the frontal lobes (Fig.
4–4). The Russian neurologist A.R. Luria demonstrated that patients
with frontal lobe injuries often lose their goal-oriented behavior.
This observation implies that when the dorsolateral frontal lobe is
injured, it cannot supply information about future goals and motives
to the temporal-parietal region. In the absence of this information,
people may not correctly perform triage or incoming sensory information and may not attend to important stimuli.

A phylogenetically older part of the brain, found in all mam-
mals, called the *limbic system*, may also be important in the triage
process. Whereas the sensory areas of the brain in the temporal,
parietal, and occipital lobes monitor the external world, through
hearing, touch, and vision, the limbic system monitors the inner
world of the body. The limbic system is also important in mediating
emotions such as fear. The portions of the brain that comprise the
limbic system are widely distributed in the brain. To influence behavior, this system has to communicate with the other neural systems. The part of the limbic system located in the middle of each
hemisphere is called the *cingulate gyrus* (Fig. 4–5). It has strong connections with the dorsolateral frontal lobes and the temporal and
parietal lobes. Patients with terminal cancer who are in severe pain
sometimes have an operation in which the neurosurgeon removes
part of the cingulate gyrus. Afterward, when these patients are asked
if they still have pain, they often answer, "Yes, but I do not pay as
much attention to the pain as I did before surgery."

The cingulate gyrus may also be injured by stroke and tumors.
When Ed Valenstein and I were searching for patients who had neglect due to frontal lesions, we found several patients with neglect
from lesions that had injured the cingulate gyrus. However, natu-
rally occurring lesions often involve more than one structure. To
determine if the cingulate gyrus was the area critical for inducing
neglect, we removed it surgically from one side of monkeys' brains

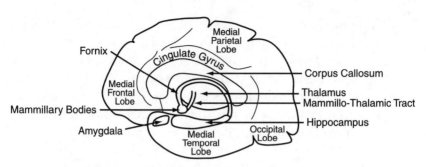

Figure 4–5. Diagram of a midsagittal section in which the brain is cut in half from front to back. This diagram shows the corpus callosum, the major connection between the right and left hemispheres. Above the corpus callosum is the cingulate gyrus.

and found that these monkeys did neglect stimuli on the opposite side of space.

Barbara Haws, our chief technician, not only took excellent care of our monkeys, but also spent so much time caring for them that she was able to make several interesting observations. Our monkeys had large homes that included a fenced-in but open area. Rural north Florida has many snakes. While some are poisonous, most are harmless. The fences, however, prevented the snakes from entering the monkeys' homes, and none were bitten. Yet Barbara noticed that when these monkeys were in the open area and saw a snake beyond the fence, they panicked. Many of our monkeys are born in captivity. Unlike people, who have language, monkeys cannot communicate verbally. Therefore, their mothers cannot tell them, "Watch out for snakes because, if they bite, you can get sick or even die." We are uncertain how these monkeys know that snakes may be dangerous. This information may be inherited rather than learned, and much inherited information that is associated with fear (fight or flight) is stored in the limbic system. After removing the cingulate gyrus on one side of a monkey's brain, my colleague Bob Watson brought a plastic snake to the laboratory. When he stood on the same side of the monkey as the injured hemisphere (nonneglected side) and wiggled the snake, the monkey panicked, but when he stood on the side of the monkey opposite the injured cingulate gyrus and wiggled the snake, the monkey showed no signs of fear. It did not panic because the cingulate gyrus, which is part of the limbic system, was injured on one side, and this injury caused the monkey to neglect the snake.

In both monkeys and humans, neglect can be caused by injury to the dorsolateral frontal lobe, the cingulate gyrus, or the inferior parietal lobe. These three areas are highly interconnected and together form a network that mediates spatially directed attention. Based on the information it receives, the parietal lobe acts like a triage officer. During a disaster, after the triage officer decides if an injured victim is immediate, delayed, expectant, or minimal, he or she must label the victim so that the treating physicians and surgeons can work on or process those labeled "immediate." The human brain separates attended from unattended stimuli by knowing the type of stimulus (what) and its location in the environment (where). To allocate attention correctly, the human inferior parietal lobe must receive this "what" and "where" information. Studies of patients with injuries to the superior portion of the parietal lobe (Fig. 4–6) reveal that they have trouble locating objects in space. For example, they may get lost when using a well-known route, or when they try to grasp or point to an object, they may miss it. These patients, however, can recognize objects. These observations suggest that the superior portion of the parietal lobe is important in determining the spatial location of objects (the "where" system) but is not important for recognizing objects (the "what" system).

In contrast to injuries of the superior parietal lobe, bilateral injuries or lesions in the inferior portion of the occipital and temporal lobes (Fig. 4–7) produce a condition call *visual object agnosia* (*a*, without; *gnosis*, knowledge). These individuals may be able to see

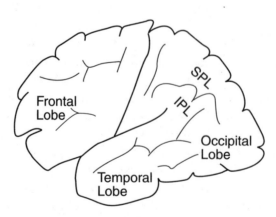

Figure 4–6. Diagram of the superior parietal lobe (SPL), which is dorsal to the inferior parietal lobe (IPL).

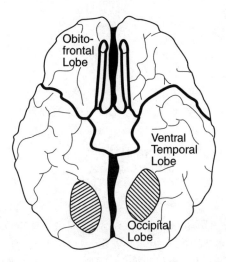

Figure 4–7. Diagram of the ventral view of the brain demonstrating the location of brain injuries associated with visual agnosia.

clearly, but they cannot recognize objects or people. At the National Institutes of Health, Leslie Ungerleider and Mortimer Mishkin studied the visual system of monkeys and observed that after nerve impulses from visual stimuli enter the primary visual cortex, in the occipital lobe, they are analyzed and processed by two visual streams. One stream goes to the parietal lobe and is called the *dorsal stream.* The other goes to the ventral temporal lobe and is called the *ventral stream* (Fig. 4–8). As observed in humans, the ventral stream, the "what" system, is important in recognizing objects, and the dorsal stream, the "where" system, is important in determining spatial location. In monkeys, the "what" and "where" systems converge in the banks of the posterior portion of the superior temporal gyrus. This region also receives input from the dorsolateral frontal lobe (goal-oriented system) and the cingulate gyrus (motivational system). Many scientists believe that the banks of the monkey's posterior superior temporal sulcus evolved into human's inferior parietal lobe (Fig. 4–9). When our group of researchers in Gainesville destroyed both banks of the posterior portion of the superior temporal gyrus, they produced the same type of neglect that is seen in humans with inferior parietal lesions.

When a person attends to an important stimulus, he or she becomes more alert or aroused. When we were doing research on

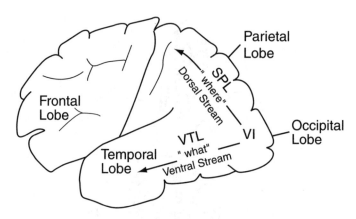

Figure 4–8. Diagram of the lateral view of the brain demonstrating the primary visual area (VI) branching into the ventral visual stream in the ventral temporal lobe (VTL), and the dorsal visual stream in the superior parietal lobe (SPL). Whereas the ventral stream mediates the "what" system, which is important in recognizing objects and people, the dorsal stream mediates the "where" system, which is important in recognizing spatial location.

the brain mechanisms of attention and neglect, Bob Watson and I saw a patient who had severe neglect of the left side of space. This deficit occurred suddenly, suggesting that the man had suffered a stroke. Because the neglect was severe, we thought the stroke had destroyed both the dorsolateral frontal lobe and the inferior parietal lobe of the right hemisphere. A CT scan of his brain, however, revealed no injury to either the frontal or the parietal lobe. Even the cerebral cortex was intact. Instead, he had a hemorrhage deep in the brain (Fig. 4–10), on the right side, in an area called the *reticular activating system*. Such hemorrhages are seen in patients with a long history of hypertension. As we mentioned in Chapter 3, about 50 years ago, Moruzzi and Magoun studied the reticular activating system in cats that were made sleepy by drugs. Using electrodes, they stimulated neurons in this activating system. On stimulation, the sleepy cats became aroused and alert. Based on these and subsequent studies, neuroscientists believe that the reticular activating system is important in arousing the brain. Physicians have learned that in people with diseases such as kidney or liver failure, toxins can accumulate and poison this area of the brain. Brain swelling can compress the reticular activating system, and drugs may poison it. Patients with these diseases first become inattentive, and as the toxin or swelling builds up, they grow less alert or even sleepy. Doctors

Human

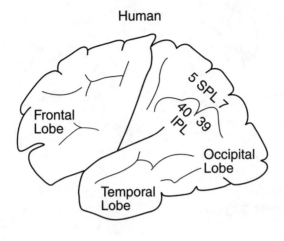

Monkey

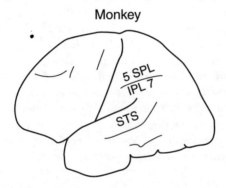

Figure 4–9. Diagrams of the lateral view of the brain in the human and the old world (rhesus) monkey. In the human brain, the inferior parietal lobe (IPL) contains two evolutionary new gyri (mounds of brain tissue) which are not found in the monkey's brain: the supramarginal gyrus (40) and the angular gyrus (39). In the monkey's brain, the IPL contains a pattern of nerve cells that the anatomist Brodmann classified as Area 7. In the human, this same area is now located in the superior parietal lobe (SPL) because of the growth of the supramarginal and angular gyri. These new gryi probably evolved from the banks of the superior temporal sulcus (STS) of non-human primates.

call this condition *delirium*. Unless it is treated, patients can slip into a coma and die.

When nerves cells send messages, they give off small electrical currents, which can be amplified and measured with an EEG. A physician who is concerned that a patient may be having epileptic seizure may order an EEG. Electroencephalography can also be used to measure brain arousal. Normally, the EEG records waves of elec-

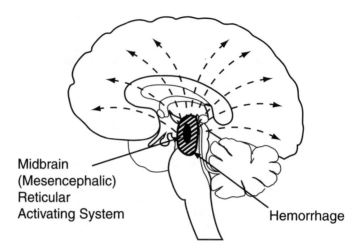

Midbrain
(Mesencephalic)
Reticular
Activating System   Hemorrhage

Figure 4–10. Diagram of a sagittal (midline) section through the brain. Under the cerebral hemispheres is an area called the *midbrain* or *mesencephalon*. The midbrain contains a large group of nerve cells called the *reticular activating system.* The reticular activating formation is located on both sides of the midbrain. The cells in this area are important in activating the higher portions of the brain including the cerebral cortex (broken lines with arrows). Stimulation of the reticular activating system arouses a sleepy animal, and injury to both sides of this system causes coma from which a person cannot be awakened. This diagram also demonstrates the position of a hemorrhage that injured the right side of the reticular formation. This lesion caused the right hemisphere to be unaroused and produced severe left-sided neglect.

trical currents. In general, the more rapid the rate of wave action, the greater the arousal. Moruzzi and Magoun recorded EEGs in cats when they stimulated the reticular activating system (Fig. 3–3 and 4–10) and found that the cats not only became alert with stimulation, but their EEG waves also became more rapid. When Bob Watson and I reviewed this classic paper, we noted something interesting about which Moruzzi and Magoun did not comment. When they stimulated the cats' reticular activating system on one side, the EEG recorded from the same side of the brain showed more arousal (the brain waves became more rapid) than did the EEG recorded from the opposite side of the brain. This suggested to us that if the reticular activating system on one side was injured, that side of the brain might become unaroused, or comatose, and unable to process stimuli from the opposite side of space.

To test this hypothesis, we made small lesions on one side of monkeys' reticular activating systems (Fig. 4–10). Postoperatively, these animals demonstrated the most severe neglect we have ever seen. We performed EEGs and found that the EEG rhythms recorded from the hemisphere with the reticular lesion were very slow.

Normally, we become aroused because there is an important stimulus in a particular area of space. Stimulus relevance is determined in part by the frontal–cingulate–parietal network we have discussed. Several investigators have stimulated different areas of the cerebral cortex to see which ones induce the greatest degree of arousal. They found that the cortical areas that influence arousal most intensely are the dorsolateral frontal lobes, the cingulate gyrus, and the parietal lobes. These are the same areas that we believe are critical in making attentional computations. Based on this set of observations, we proposed that a cortical–frontal-parietal–limbic (cingulate)–reticular network is important in mediating attention to stimuli on the opposite side of space (Fig. 4–11).

Right–Left Asymmetries of Attention

Many neurologists have noted that in patients with unilateral neglect, the lesion is much more likely to occur in the right hemisphere. Some have thought that it might only appear that neglect is more commonly associated with right-sided brain damage because patients with large lesions in the left hemisphere may be aphasic and unable to comprehend speech or reading, so that they cannot be adequately tested. Even when using nonverbal tasks without verbal

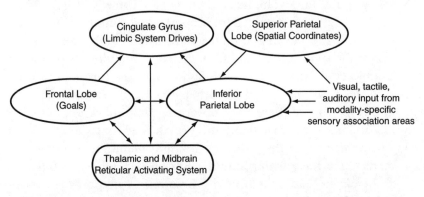

Figure 4–11. Diagram of the cortical (frontal and parietal)–limbic (cingulate gyrus)–reticular network, which is important in mediating attention.

instructions, however, several investigators have found that neglect is both more common and more severe with right than with left hemisphere lesions. To account for this asymmetry, we suggested that perhaps the left hemisphere attends to stimuli primarily on the right side of the body and head, whereas the right hemisphere attends to stimuli in both left and right hemispace. Therefore, if the left hemisphere is injured, severe neglect does not occur because the right hemisphere can attend to ipsilateral right hemispace. However, when the right hemisphere is injured, the left hemisphere can attend to the right but not the left side of space, and the patient is inattentive to or unaware of stimuli in left space.

To test this hypothesis, Tom Van Den Abell and I studied normal college students with EEG, attaching electrodes to the area of the scalp over the right and left parietal lobes. The subjects sat at a table on which there was an apparatus with three lights. This apparatus was placed about 3 feet in front of the subject so that the middle light was directly in front of the subject's nose, the right light was in front of the subject's right ear, and the left light was in front of the subject's left ear. Directly in front of the subject's chest, we also placed a telegraph key. We told the subjects that their job was to press the telegraph key as soon as possible after they saw the middle light come on. We also told them that the lights on the right or left side might come on a little before the middle light and act as a warning that the middle light was going to come on.

The time period between the middle light coming on and the subject pushing the telegraph key is called the *reaction time.* Runners and swimmers know that if, before the starting gun goes off, a warning is given ("Take your mark, get set . . ."), they will get off the starting block more rapidly than if no warning stimulus is provided. One reason the warning stimulus reduces reaction time is that it instructs the subject to attend to the starting stimulus. As predicted, our subjects' reaction times were faster when the turning on of the middle light was preceded by either a right or left-sided warning stimulus than when there was no warning stimulus. The EEG taken while subjects were performing this task showed that when the warning stimulus was on the left side, the right hemisphere became activated. When the warning stimulus was on the right side, however, both hemispheres were activated. These results support the hypothesis that whereas the left hemisphere attends primarily to stimuli on the right side, the right hemisphere attends to stimuli on both sides. Therefore, if a person has a stroke in the left hemisphere, the right hemisphere can still attend to the right side of space, but if the stroke affects the right hemisphere, the left hemisphere can attend only to the right side of space; the left side of space goes unattended.

Several years after our report of this experiment was published in *Neurology*, I went to a scientific meeting where a neuroscientist presented a functional imaging study. In this study, the researchers injected radioisotopes into subjects. The radioisotopes went to the active areas of the brain. The researchers used this technique to learn which areas of the brain are activated during an attentional task. They found that when the left side was stimulated, only the right hemisphere was activated, but when the right side was stimulated, both hemispheres were activated, suggesting that the left hemisphere attends to the right side of space and the right hemisphere attends to both the right and the left sides. The neuroscientist who presented this paper also mentioned that some investigators in a remote little southern town using EEG had described a similar observation.

When I first moved to this "remote little southern town" called Gainesville, it took me only 10 minutes to drive from my home to the hospital. As the town grew and traffic got worse, the trip began to take 20 or even 30 minutes. I am one of those people who constantly talks to themselves, especially when heavy traffic makes driving slow. On the way to work one morning, I was speculating about why the brain was designed so that the left hemisphere attends to the right side of space and the right hemisphere attends to both sides. Just then, a car on my right side drove through a stop sign without stopping. I immediately attended to this car, swerved, and just missed being hit. After calming down, I started ruminating again and then realized why the brain might have this hemispheric attentional asymmetry. Since the left hemisphere mediates speech-language, when a person is talking the left hemisphere cannot be vigilant for stimuli on the right, but because the right hemisphere can attend to both sides of space, it can attend to cars on the right while the left hemisphere is busy talking. Specialization permits parallel processing.

SPOTLIGHTS AND FLOODLIGHTS OF ATTENTION

Evelyn George was born and raised on a ranch just south of Saint Mary's River, which separates eastern Florida from eastern Georgia. She rarely saw doctors. Once when she was in a pharmacy in Jacksonville, buying inexpensive reading glasses, store personnel were checking customers' blood pressures. Her blood pressure was found to be 200/120. The young woman who took her blood pressure was so alarmed that she took it again and found that it was about the same. She told Mrs. George that her blood pressure was very high and that she needed to see a doctor as soon as possible. Driving in Jacksonville made Mrs. George nervous. She did not have a family doctor, had no insurance, and did not follow this advice. Several weeks after her blood pressure was taken in the pharmacy, she drove her old pickup truck down to a farm outside of Gainesville to visit her son and granddaughter. After dinner, she sat down on the couch to watch television and seemed to doze off. When her son had the coffee ready, he tried to wake her but had trouble doing so. When she finally opened her eyes, she seemed confused. He called 911.

When the paramedics arrived they took her blood pressure, which was now 230/150. They transported her to Shands Hospital at the University of Florida, where she was admitted and sent to the intensive care unit (ICU) to receive intravenous drugs to reduce her blood pressure. The doctors thought her high blood pressure was causing her confusion, a condition called *hypertensive encephalopathy* (*encephalo* brain; *pathy*, sick). However, when her blood pressure returned to the normal range, she still appeared confused. The doctors then thought that she might have suffered an intracerebral hemorrhage, one of the most serious complications of severe hypertension. They performed a CT brain scan, which showed no hemorrhage but did show two cerebral infarctions, one in the superior parietal lobe of each hemisphere (Fig. 4–12). Severe hypertension often causes the blood vessels in the brain to go into spasm, which prevents them from bringing sufficient blood to areas of the brain. The doctors in the ICU called for a neurology consultation, and the patient was transferred to the neurology service.

Bob Watson, the attending neurologist, noted that Mrs. George's main problem involved visual recognition and asked me to examine her in our weekly neurology grand rounds. When I tested her visual acuity it seemed excellent, as she was able to read quite small letters. To see if she had lost vision in a specific spatial sector, I had her fix her eyes on my nose while I wiggled my finger in different areas of space and asked her to point to my finger when it moved. She performed flawlessly. Then I asked her to touch my finger with her index finger. She had trouble with this simple task,

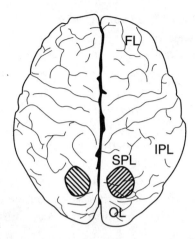

Figure 4–12. Diagram of Mrs. George's CT scan showing two cerebral in-farctions (strokes), one in the left superior parietal lobe (SPL) and the other in the right superior parietal lobe (FL = frontal lobe, OL = occipital lobe, IPL = inferior parietal lobe).

often missing my finger. This reaching disorder is called *optic ataxia*. It is caused by lesions in the parietal lobes that extend deep into subcortical structures. The cerebral cortex, or gray matter, contains the nerve cells and the short connections between them. Under the cortex (subcortical region) is the white matter of the brain. The subcortical region contains axons that resemble electrical wires com-ing from the bodies of nerve cells situated in the cerebral cortex. These axons connect one area of the brain with others. Geschwind thought that parietal lobe lesions caused optic ataxia because they prevented visual information, which comes from the occipital lobes situated in the posterior part of the brain, from reaching the motor neurons located in the posterior portion of the frontal lobes. With-out this visual information, the motor cortex cannot correctly con-trol arm movements.

There is, however, another explanation for optic ataxia. Re-search in monkeys and humans suggests that the region of the pa-rietal cortex where Mrs. George's infarctions occurred is important for spatial analysis. The spatial analysis performed by the parietal lobes might be similar to analyses students perform on graph paper when they take a course in analytic geometry. To graph the position of an object in space in relation to your body, you may want to use a three-dimensional grid with three axes: horizontal (right to left), vertical (up and down), and radial (front to back). The region directly in front of your eyes could be the area where all three axes meet. This is called the *zero point*. An object to the right of your midline might be given a positive value, and an object to the left a negative value. Similarly, if an object is above or in front of your zero point it would have a positive value, and if below or behind it, it would have a negative value. In this graph, if each unit equaled 1 inch and an object's position had coordinates of -30, $+ 40$, and $+20$, this would mean that the object is 30 inches to the left of midline, 40 inches above eye level, and 20 inches in front of your eyes. Some investigators believe that when you see an object in space, it is the parietal lobes that compute these coordinates and then supply this information to other regions of the brain, such as the motor areas that are important in programming movements of the arms. If this part of the brain is injured, as it was in Mrs. George, the individual cannot compute the locations of objects in space and thus has optic ataxia.

Mrs. George also had difficulty moving her eyes (*ocular ataxia* or *psychic paralysis of gaze*) to fixate on the target at which she wanted to gaze. Like the hands and arms, the eyes are directed by a motor system. The motor system that controls eye movements is independent of the motor system that controls arm movements, but this oculo-motor system also relies on the computations of the spatial coordinate system that was injured in this woman.

Although Mrs. George had optic ataxia, once her eyes found the object she was able to continue to gaze at it. She could name objects I showed her, but when I presented a picture of a family eating dinner and asked her to describe it, she said it was a picture of an apple. Since her visual acuity was excellent and she could see my hands in all portions of space (normal visual fields), her response surprised me. I thought that perhaps she did not understand me, so I asked her again to tell me what the picture was illustrating. She turned, looked at me, looked back at the picture, and again said, "This is a picture of an apple. See, here is the apple." She then pointed to an apple on the table in the picture but ignored the rest of the picture. Someone who was attending grand rounds found another complex picture. This was a painting of a Civil War battle. It looked like the Battle of Olustee, which took place very close to Mrs. George's home. She looked at the picture and said, "This is a picture of a bird." She then pointed to a bird that the artist had placed above the battle scene. "See here, there is the bird that is flying." She never mentioned anything else.

This disorder, in which the person sees only a small part of a complex picture, is called *simultanagnosia* (*simultan* = simultaneous; *a* = without; *gnosia* = knowledge). The combination of simultanagnosia, optic ataxia, and ocular ataxia is called *Balint's syndrome*, named after the neurologist who first described it in 1909. The mechanism that accounts for the inability to see the whole picture is not known. For some tasks, we need a narrow focus of attention, or spotlight; for others, we need a broad view, or floodlight. See Figure 4–13 for an example of a task that may require a floodlight or a spotlight. Although a floodlight and a spotlight may have equal wattage, the lens on the spotlight focuses light in a small area and the lens on the floodlight distributes light to a large area. Anna Barrett and other investigators in our laboratory have found that the parietal lobe is important in controlling how narrowly or widely attention should be focused for a specific task. Perhaps Mrs. George couldn't use her attentional floodlight, depended on her attentional spotlight, and missed the "big picture."

The Navon figure in Figure 4–13 is designed to pit these two attentional lenses against each other. If you look at this figure and first see the letter *H*, this might suggest that you tend to use your attentional floodlight first. In contrast, if you see the letter *A* first, this might suggest that you tend to use your attentional spotlight. After giving patients with unilateral brain damage a similar task, Lynn Robertson and her coworkers found that whereas the left hemi-

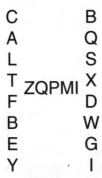

Figure 4–13. Navon figure. A Patient who has a problem with the attentional floodlight may be unable to find the large letter *H*. A patient who has a problem with the attentional spotlight may be unable to find the letter *A*.

sphere is important in mediating the spotlight, the right hemisphere is important in mediating the floodlight.

HABITUATION

When you were reminded about your left foot you may have attended to it and felt it for a few minutes, but before you started reading this section you may have again become unaware of that foot. You became unaware of it because there were no novel stimuli impinging on it and nothing was happening to it that needed your attention. The phenomenon of becoming unaware of irrelevant stimuli is called *habituation*. You can habituate in all sensory modalities. For example, when you walk into a room to read, you may hear the air conditioner and smell an odor, but a few minutes after you start to read, you may no longer be aware of them.

While testing Mrs. George's vision I observed another defect that I'd never seen before. I held up a pen and asked her what it was. She responded, "It's a pen." The I asked her to tell me as much about the pen as she could (e.g., What kind of pen is it? What are its colors? Does it have a clip?). She then said, "Dr. Heilman, I know this sounds funny, but I cannot see the pen. It disappeared." I thought something had happened to her vision. Perhaps another stroke had destroyed her primary visual areas, so I put the pen down because I wanted to examine her vision further. When I moved the pen, she said, "There, now that you moved the pen, I can see it again." I didn't know if her visual cortex was temporarily deprived of blood or if this phenomenon was a result of her previous stroke. To continue the test, I held up my keys and asked her to stare at them. After a few seconds she said, "The keys disappeared." When I moved the keys, she said, "There they are again." I asked how long she had been having this problem with disappearing objects. She said, "Since I had my stroke, but I didn't tell because I am worried that the doctors would think that I'm crazy."

Mark Mennemeier, a postdoctoral fellow in our laboratory at that time, told me that this phenomenon of objects disappearing can even be seen in normal people. For example, if you look at the cross on the right side of Figure 4–14, at first you will see the dot on the left side of the page. However, if you keep staring at the cross without moving you eyes or the paper, after about 20 to 30 seconds the dot will either fade or disappear. This fading phenomenon in

Figure 4–14. If you stare at the X on the right side of the page without moving your eyes or the page, after about 30 to 60 seconds the dot on the left side of the page may either disappear or fade. This phenomenon is called *sensory habituation.* After the dot fades, if you move the page it will reappear.

normal people is called the *Troxler effect.* If you move either your eyes or the paper, the dot will reappear. What was abnormal about Mrs. George was that the disappearing items were in her central vision, and they disappeared very rapidly.

In the center or core of the brain is a sensory relay structure called the *thalamus* (Fig. 4–15). Sensory information coming from the visual, auditory, and tactile systems must pass through the thalamus before entering the cerebral cortex for analysis. Each of the sensory systems courses through a different area of the thalamus.

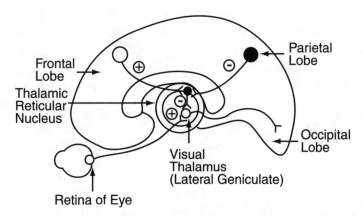

Figure 4–15. Diagram of the thalamus, which is located below the cortex in the center of each hemisphere. On the onside, surrounding the thalamus, is a group of nerves called the *thalamic reticular nucleus.* These cells normally inhibit visual (or other sensory) stimuli from traveling to the cerebral cortex for further processing. The parietal lobes appear to inhibit (−) these inhibitory cells and the frontal lobes activate (+) these inhibitory thalamic reticular neurons, thereby blocking the transmission of sensory information to the cerebral cortex. In this figure the inhibitory cells (−) are dark and the excitatory cells (+) are light.

Surrounding these areas of the sensory thalamus is a neural structure called the *thalamic reticular nucleus.* This structure has nerve cells
that project to the sensory relay areas of the thalamus. The thalamic
reticular nerves are inhibitory and, when activated, they prevent the
thalamic sensory areas from transmitting sensory information to the
cortex. Therefore, the thalamus is not only a relay station but also
may be a gate that controls which sensory information reaches to
the cerebral cortex. Based on our observations of Mrs. George, we
proposed that areas of the cerebral cortex may control this sensory
gate, either opening or closing it. That objects disappeared rapidly
for Mrs. George suggests that her sensory gate was closing prema-
turely. Since she had parietal lobe lesions, we proposed that normally the parietal lobes may open the gate by inhibiting this inhibitory thalamic reticular nucleus. We also thought that the frontal
lobes might be important for closing this gate. To test this hypothesis, Mark Mennemeier and others in our laboratory used the Troxler test with patients who had frontal and parietal lesions. Our findings support this hypothesis. One patient, with a parietal lesion in
one hemisphere and a frontal lesion in the other hemisphere, was
particularly interesting. Using a Troxler fading test, we found that
when the dot was on the side of space opposite the parietal lobe
lesion, the patient experienced fading more rapidly than did control
subjects. When the dot was on the side of space opposite the frontal
lobe lesion, fading took much longer than it did in the controls or
did not occur. These observations indicate that whereas the parietal
lobes are important in helping us attend to novel or important stimuli, the frontal lobes are important in helping us withdraw attention
from insignificant stimuli.

SUMMARY

The brain has a limited processing capacity and receives more information than it can process fully. We attend to stimuli that are
important and ignore those that are unimportant. Stimulus significance is determined by our immediate needs (drives) and future
goals. When the inferior parietal lobe, the dorsolateral frontal lobe,
or the cingulate gyrus is injured, patients are inattentive to stimuli
on the opposite side of space. In addition to receiving projections
from the sensory association cortex (visual, auditory, and tactile),

the inferior parietal lobe has reciprocal projections with the dorsolateral frontal lobe and the cingulate gyrus. The frontal lobes are
important in mediating goal-oriented behavior and the cingulate
gyrus, a portion of the limbic system, is important in mediating
drives and emotional behaviors. Thus, a frontal lobe–cingulate gyrus–inferior parietal lobe network is critical in determining stimulus
significance. When a person attends to an important stimulus, he or
she becomes more alert or aroused. Arousal increases the brain's
processing capacity. The midbrain (mesencephalon) contains a
group of neurons called the reticular activating system, which when
stimulated produces cortical activation or arousal. The dorsolateral
frontal lobe, the cingulate gyrus, and the parietal lobe control this
activating system. The cortical–(frontal-parietal)–limbic (cingulate)–
reticular network, important in mediating attention-arousal, is summarized in Figure 4–11. Although each hemisphere contains one of
these networks, the network in the right hemisphere appears to be
dominant. In addition, some tasks require us to focus attention on
a small area of space (attentional spotlight), and other tasks require
us to attend to a large area of space (attentional floodlight). Studies
of patients with posterior temporal-inferior parietal lesions suggest
that the left hemisphere may be more important for focused attention and the right for distributed attention. Finally we become unaware of irrelevant stimuli (habituation). The frontal lobes might be
important in closing the gate in the thalamus, thereby preventing
stimuli from reach in cerebral cortex, and the parietal lobe might
be important in opening this gate.

Selected Readings

De Renzi, E (1982) *Disorders of space exploration and cognition*, Wiley,
New York.

Heilman, K.M., Watson, R.T., Valenstein, E. (1993) Neglect and related disorders. In *Clinical neuropsychology*, Heilman, K.M. and
Valenstein E. University Press, Oxford, New York, pp. 279–336.

Heilman, K.M., Valenstein, E, Watson, R.T. (1983) Localization of
neglect. In *Localization in neurology*. (Ed.) Kertesz A. Academic
Press, New York, pp. 471–492.

Jeannerod, M. (1987) *Neurophysiological and neuropsychological aspects
of spatial neglect.* Elsevier, Amsterdam.

Pardo, J.V., Fox, P.T., and Raichle, M.E. (1991) Localization of a

human system for sustained attention by positron emission tomography. *Nature* 349:61–64.

Posner, M.I., and Rafal, R.D. (1987). Cognitive theories of attention
and rehabilitation of attentional deficits. In *Neuropsychological rehabilitation*, (Ed.) Mier, M.J., and Benton, A.L., and Diller, L.
Guilford Press, New York, pp. 182–201

Roberson, I.H., Marshall, J.C., (1993) *Unilateral neglect: Clinical and
experimental studies.* Lawerence Erlbaum, Hove, United Kingdom.

CHAPTER

5

SELF-AWARENESS

In *Webster's International Dictionary* the word *consciousness* has nine different definitions. One of the definitions is "knowing or perceiving something within oneself or a fact about oneself." This chapter will discuss the brain mechanisms that are important for self-knowledge. It is called "Self-Awareness" rather than "Consciousness" because the other forms of consciousness, such as being alert and awake rather than unconscious, are not discussed here.

ASOMATOGNOSIA: A DEFICIT OF SELF-KNOWLEDGE

One way to approach the brain mechanisms of self-awareness is to study patients who have lost this capacity. In the previous chapter, I told the story of George Jones, who had hemispatial neglect and was aware of only the right side of his food tray. Several days after I turned his food tray so that he could find the meat, he again called me over to his bed. "Hey, Doc, over here." When I came over to his bed, he lifted his weak left arm with his right arm and asked, me, "Could you get this guy out of my bed?" I was surprised by his request and thought that I might have not heard him correctly, so I asked, "Could you repeat that?" He said, "Yes! I want this person out of my bed." I told him that the arm he was holding was his own. He said, "You know, it looks like my arm, but it does not belong to me." I then tried to show him that the hand he was lifting was connected to a wrist, the wrist was connected to a forearm, the forearm was connected to an arm, the arm was connected to a shoulder, and the shoulder was attached to his chest. Still, I could not convince him that this arm was his own. After walking away from his bed to see another patient, I noticed that he had lifted his left hand with the right and tried to throw it out of bed. Because of his stroke, however, his arm was spastic. Muscles in a spastic arm act like a spring, so that when he tried to throw his arm out of the bed, it just sprang back and hit him in the chest. After doing this several times he said, "You see, this guy will not get out of my bed."

During our neurology training in Boston, my friend and colleague Ed Valenstein told me about one of his patients with a similar problem due to a large right hemisphere stroke. When this man rolled over in bed so that his right side was toward the mattress, he asked Dr. Valenstein who was lying on top of him. Soon after arriving at the University of Florida, I took care of a young woman, the wife of one of our medical residents, who had developed unilateral neglect after a cerebral hemorrhage in her right hemisphere. When she came to the hospital, the nurses dressed her in a hospital gown and helped her into bed. Then she rubbed her right thigh against her left. She giggled, blushed, and asked, "Who is in bed with me?"

This inability to recognize one side of the body as belonging to oneself is called *asomatognosia* (*a* = without, *somato* = body, *gnosia* = knowledge). Asomatognosia is often, but not always, associated with spatial neglect. I returned to Mr. Jones's bedside and told him that the arm he was throwing out of bed was his own. I also told him that the reason the arm felt as if it did not belong to him was that it was weak and numb.

I was worried that Mr. Jones would become frustrated or hurt himself by continually trying to throw his left arm out of bed, but I did not know what else to do. On rounds the next day, I told Dr. Fritz Dreyfus, Professor of Neurology, about his behavior and asked him how we could help Mr. Jones. He said, "Lightly restrain his left arm to the left side of the bed." I asked, "Wouldn't that be uncomfortable for him?" He answered, "No, it will not. As far as he is concerned, it is not his left arm. Remember that he also has unilateral spatial neglect and is unaware of objects on his left side, so once you get the arm into his left space, he will be unaware that it is restrained."

Later that morning, I went to see Mr. Jones and asked him if he still wanted me to get his arm out of bed. He said, "Yes, I do not want this person in my bed." I gently picked up his arm and strapped it loosely to the left side of the bed. After his arm was moved off his chest he said, "Thanks, Doc, I do not know what that guy was doing in my bed." Later that morning, Mr. Jones called me over to his bed again and said, "Doc, I think this guy you took out of bed this morning may be holding me down." I asked if he would rather have that arm in bed with him or held down. He said, "Neither." I told him that I would release his left arm from the restraint so that he could roll over, and as he got better he would realize that the arm he thought belonged to someone else was really his.

Although most patients with asomatognosia have an injury to the right parietal lobe, the mechanism underlying this defect is not entirely understood. The two mechanisms that have been suggested to account for this dramatic sign are impaired sensory feedback and a defect in body image, or self-representational disorder. I will briefly discuss each of these possible mechanisms.

Normally, information about our limbs' position in space is constantly being fed back to the brain. Injury to a hemisphere may prevent this information from being received and interpreted. Like Mr. Jones, many patients with asomatognosia have hemineglect, or unawareness of stimuli on the left side of space and on the left side of the body. Many also have severe left–sided weakness or hemiplegia. The knowledge that something exists is based on experiencing or perceiving that entity. If a person's arm is paralyzed, has no feeling, and is not experienced by normal parts of the brain, perhaps that person becomes unaware of its existence. To learn if this sensory feedback deficit could account for asomatoagnosia, we tested patients whose right hemisphere was put asleep as a result of selective barbiturate anesthesia (the Wada test). We put a hemisphere to sleep when we are evaluating patients for possible neurosurgery. Some patients with severe epilepsy, whose seizures cannot be controlled by medicines, may benefit from surgical removal of part of the brain. We use this test to make certain that we do not remove areas of the brain that are important for speech and memory. During the time when the right hemisphere is asleep, some patients develop asomatognosia. To learn if asomatognosia was caused by an absence of sensory feedback, we wrote a number on the patients' palms and on the examiner's palm, moved the patients' or examiner's palm to the patients' right side, where it could be seen, and asked the patients to read the number. We performed this procedure to demonstrate that the patients had sensory (visual) feedback. If they could read the number, we then asked them to tell us if the hand that was being shown to them was their hand or the examiner's hand. Despite this visual feedback, many of these patients did not recognize their own hand (asomatognosia). Although this observation suggests that asomatognosia is not caused by a total absence of sensory feedback, it remains possible that somatosensory feedback (e.g., touch and position) is more important than visual feedback for developing the experience of ownership.

Several investigators in the early twentieth century thought that the brain contains representations or memories of the body. Because the left side of the body is represented in the right hemisphere's parietal lobe, injury to the right parietal lobe destroys these memories and patients are unaware that their left side belongs to them. Several observations support this representational hypothesis.

Although I did not directly observe Mr. Jones dressing, the nurses told the doctors that his wife brought his pajamas to the hospital so that he did not have to wear the hospital gowns that most patients seem to detest. After he had his morning bath, a nursing student gave him his pajamas and he attempted to put them on. The nursing student went to the bathroom to dispose of the dirty bath water and to clean the wash basin, but when she returned to his bedside, she was surprised to learn that he had dressed only his right side. Only his right leg was in the pajama bottoms, and only his right arm was in the top. The left half of the body remained nude. When she asked him why he dressed only the right side of his body, he seemed to be unaware that there was any problem with his dressing. Although the unawareness that his left side was nude could be explained by defective sensory feedback, his failure to know that there was a left side to dress could not result from a sensory deficit, but rather suggests a body image or representational deficit.

The hypothesis that asomatognosia is caused by a representational deficit of the body image is supported by the phantom limb phenomenon. After a body part is lost or removed, some people feel that it is still present. This feeling is called a *phantom*, and the best-known type is the phantom limb. I saw my first case as an intern on a rotation in the Memorial Sloan-Kettering Cancer Center. Judy Margolin was a 19-year-old woman who had a bone cancer (sarcoma) of her left arm. To stop the spread of this cancer, the surgeons amputated her arm and shoulder. After this surgery, she was transferred to our medical service because she was receiving radiation therapy and chemotherapy, which often make patients weak and sick. Judy's major problem, however, was not generalized weakness or nausea and vomiting, but pain. At that time, I did not know that she had phantom limb pain. She only told me that she had pain in the area of the operation. Unfortunately, I never asked her about phantom pain. Antidepressant medication, often used successfully to treat pain, was not available then. Although anticonvulsants such as Dilantin, which are used to treat epilepsy, were available, we did not know then that these could be used to treat pain. Because Judy was suffering so much, I tried strong pain killers such as morphine. These medicines reduced her suffering somewhat, but she continued to have pain. Someone mentioned to me that there is a doctor in physical medicine at New York University who was an expert in treating this type of pain. Because we were part of the Cornell University Medical Center, I had to get permission for this doctor to see Judy. Fortunately, once I told the administrators about this patient, permission was granted and this kind physician came to see Judy the same day I called. After examining her surgical wound, he asked if she felt that her shoulder and arm were still with her. Judy said, "Yes, it feels like I still have my arm and it hurts." He said, "Please try to tell me the position of the arm in relation to your body." She said, "My hand and forearm feel like they are behind my back and someone is twisting them." At about that time, two surgeons came to Judy's room. They watched and listened to her speak with this visiting physician and seemed surprised that he was talking about something that was not there. But, apparently fascinated by the conversation, they didn't say anything. The expert then asked Judy, "Can you move the hand and forearm that is behind you?" She was silent for a few moments and then asked, "Should I try?" He nodded. She grimaced as if she was making a strong effort and then said, "Yes, but just a little." He said, "Good! I will leave a set of exercises with your nurse. I want you to exercise that arm three times a day so that we can get it into a comfortable position, and hopefully that will decrease your pain." He also told her, "Usually, after several months, the arm will feel like it is shrinking back into your body, and then your pain will be almost all gone." After this brief encounter Judy already looked better, and her need for morphine declined.

From this experience, I learned not only about phantom limbs but also about how important hope is to patients. Although one should never lie to patients, a physician also should never destroy hope.

I never learned whether these exercises worked. It was near the end of my rotation at Memorial Sloan-Kettering, and I had to move on to another hospital. Another intern who took over Judy's case told me that the surgery, radiation therapy, and chemotherapy did not stop the cancer, which spread rapidly until she died a few months later.

That people who have lost a limb remain aware of it supports the representational (body memory) hypothesis that we have discussed. Patients have the phantom limb syndrome because they still have the representation of the limb in their brains. In the opposite condition, asomatoagnosia, the brain's representation of a limb is lost and even though the limb is present, the person is unaware of it.

ANOSOGNOSIA: UNAWARENESS OF WEAKNESS

After his stroke Mr. Jones had very severe left-sided weakness, but whenever I asked him if his left arm was any better he responded, "Doctor, there is nothing wrong with my left arm." When I asked him why he was in the hospital he said, "My family brought me." When I asked why his family had brought him, he said, "They told me that I had a stroke." Then I asked how the stroke had affected him. He said, "I guess I am pretty lucky because I have no weakness and still talk, read, and write." A French neurologist, Joseph Francois Felix Babinski, was one of the first to describe this dramatic disorder almost 100 years ago. He coined the term *anosognosia* (*a* = without; *noso* = disease; *gnosia* = knowledge) to denote this unawareness of weakness on one side of a body (*hemiplegia*).

Anosognosia is not a trivial problem. If a patient comes into a hospital immediately after developing symptoms such as weakness, and the neurologist makes a diagnosis of stroke caused by a blood clot in one of the carotid arteries (a pair of large vessels that brings blood to the brain), she or he can be treated with a clot-busting drug that may reduce the severity of permanent injury. The clot-busting drug must be given less than 3 hours after stroke onset. If they are administered after 3 hours, there is a good chance that the patient will suffer a hemorrhage into the brain. Patients who are not aware that they are weak may delay seeking treatment and may be ineligible for this treatment. Mr. Jones's doctors asked that he be seen by an occupational therapist who could teach him to perform the skills that would allow him to care for himself, as well as a physical therapist who could teach him to walk and increase the strength of his weak extremities. He refused this therapy because he thought he was not weak. Another problem is that patients who do not recognize their impairment sometimes engage in activities that may harm themselves or others. They may try to drive or use heavy machinery or power tools. For example, I had a patient who was unaware of his left-sided blindness. Despite being warned about returning to work or driving, he did both. At work he was seriously injured when a crane carrying a steel beam hit the left side of his head.

Asomatognosia Hypothesis of Anosognosia

Anosognosia, like asomatognosia (unawareness of one-half of the body), is a deficit of self-awareness. Like many other patients with anosognosia, Mr. Jones had asomatognosia and even tried to throw his arm out of bed because he thought it belonged to someone else. One possible reason patients do not recognize the weakness of their left arm is that they do not recognize that their left hand and arm belong to them.

To learn if asomatognosia causes anosognosia, we studied patients who were undergoing the Wada test or selective hemispheric anesthesia. When these patients' right hemispheres were anesthetized, we showed them either their own weak left hands or the examiner's left hand. We restricted their view so that when we showed them the examiner's hand, they were unable to see their own left hands. We showed them this hand on the right side so that it could be perceived by the awake left hemisphere. Then we asked them if the hand that they were viewing was their hand or someone else's hand (a test for asomatognosia). We also asked them if they thought that their hand was weak (a test for anosognosia). Although a few patients denied having weakness (anosognosia) and were unable to recognize their own left hand (asomatoagnosia), most of those who were unaware of their weakness were able to identify their own hand. These results suggest that in most people asomatognosia cannot fully account for anosognosia. Thus, some other defect must be accounting for this deficit of self-awareness.

Psychological Denial Hypothesis of Anosognosia

About 40 years ago, Ed Weinstein and Robert Kahn wrote a book called *Denial of Illness.* In addition to providing a detailed clinical description of anosognosia, these authors proposed that this disorder is induced by psychologically motivated denial of a catastrophic event, that is, a psychological defense mechanism. To test this hypothesis, they assessed patient's personalities by interviewing their relatives and close associates. They found that patients with anosognosia more often used denial as a coping strategy before their current illness than did patients who were without anosognosia.

When I read Weinstein and Kahn's book, the idea that a patient would deny having the symptoms and signs of an illness as a defense mechanism seemed unreasonable to me. I had heard that Ed Weinstein, who was a neurologist at the Bronx Veteran's Administration Hospital, had also trained as a psychiatrist, and I suspected that he was using psychoanalytic theory to explain this neurologic disorder. In the summer of 1998, however, I played singles tennis on a hot Florida day after finishing 18 holes of golf. After the match was over, I got into my car, started retching, and had some chest pain. I thought that I had probably become overheated and that the retching was causing the pain. I drove home, and as I cooled off the retching subsided, but I still felt the chest pain. Thinking that it might be related to esophageal irritation, I took the antacid Tagamet and waited for the pain to subside. All the time I was sweating, which I ascribed to being overheated from playing tennis. After about 15 minutes the pain became worse, so I told my wife to drive me to the hospital because I might be having a heart attack. At the hospital emergency room, an electrocardiogram showed that there was no question about it: I was having a heart attack. If someone had described to me the symptoms I had experienced, I would have told them, "Call 911 immediately. You need to go to the hospital as soon as possible. You may be having a heart attack." People who know me well would also agree that one of my defense mechanisms has always been denial. When it comes to their own and their families' health, physicians often use denial. My mentor, Norman Geschwind, developed chest pains in his fifties while listening to the Boston Symphony. He went home, took a bath, and was found dead. Perhaps in medical school, when we see how many diseases can cause death, disability, and suffering, we start building a wall and deny that we and our loved ones can develop these diseases. This wall allows us to see and concentrate on the patient's problems without always thinking, "My wife, my children, or I could get this." My own experience made me realize that Weinstein and Kahn had a point: psychological denial is real, but can it entirely explain anosognosia?

When Babinski first described anosognosia in 1917, the patient he reported had a left hemiplegia from a right hemisphere stroke. Other neurologists have since observed that anosognosia is more frequently associated with right than with left hemisphere damage. The observation that anosognosia for hemiplegia is more frequently associated with right than left hemisphere injury is incompatible with the psychological denial hypothesis. Although Weinstein and Kahn were aware of these observations, they also knew that in most people language is mediated by the left hemisphere and that people with large left hemisphere strokes may be unable to deny their illness because many of them suffer a loss of language (aphasia). They therefore reasoned that anosognosia is more often reported with right than with left hemisphere lesions because it could not be assessed in patients with severe aphasia due to left hemisphere damage. According to Weinstein and Kahn, the reported hemispheric asymmetry of anosognosia did not refute their psychological denial hypothesis because this asymmetry was related to a sampling bias.

Selective hemisphere anesthesia (the Wada test) causes the contralateral arm to become weak. Finding that unawareness of weakness is more frequently associated with right than left hemisphere dysfunction would disprove the psychological denial hypothesis. To test the denial hypothesis by investigating whether hemispheric asymmetry of anosognosia exists, we first thought that we could ask epileptic patients who were being evaluated for surgery by selective right and left hemispheric anesthesia if they felt weak. During anesthesia of the language-dominant hemisphere, however, patients would be aphasic and unable to speak or comprehend. To avoid this confounding circumstance, we decided to ask this question after they recovered from the hemispheric anesthesia, and their aphasia. This study revealed that after right hemisphere but not left hemisphere anesthesia, patients were often unaware that their arm had been weak. These results did not support Weinstein and Kahn's psychological denial hypothesis for two reasons. First, if patients deny their hemiplegia because psychologically they have trouble dealing with a catastrophic event, they would not be expected to deny hemiplegia as part of a test, especially since they were asked about it after recovering from the anesthesia and weakness. Second, Weinstein and Kahn's theory cannot explain why the patients' denial is more frequently associated with anesthesia of the right than the left hemisphere.

There may be an alternative explanation of these results. It is possible that after patients recover from right hemispheric anesthesia, they do not recall that they were weak because putting this hemisphere to sleep also caused a memory deficit, but if they were asked when they were weak, they may have been aware of their weakness. Thus, the problem could be one of memory rather than unawareness. To test this idea, we asked our patients both during and after right hemispheric anesthesia if they thought their arm was weak. Those who were unaware of their arm weakness after hemispheric anesthesia were the same patients who were unaware of it during hemispheric anesthesia. The right–left differences we observed were within the same person, and the unawareness of weakness with anesthesia of one but not the other hemisphere cannot be explained by personality factors.

Using this same hemispheric anesthesia technique, we made another observation that does not support the denial theory of anosognosia. After recovering from left (dominant) hemispheric anesthesia, some patients were unaware of their right arm weakness but were aware that they could not speak properly, while other patients were unaware that they had trouble speaking (anosognosia of aphasia) but were aware of their arm weakness. The psychological denial theory does account for this dissociation. It suggests that the brain mechanisms underlying unawareness of weakness are different from the brain mechanisms underlying unawareness of aphasia.

Defective Feedback Hypothesis of Anosognosia

Unawareness of an event implies a lack of information. Another possible explanation of anosognosia for weakness is that the brain injury associated with it could have caused sensory *feedback* deficits that prevented the patient from learning that his or her arm was not working. We get feedback about the movements of our limbs from the sensory system in the limb that detects movement (proprioception) and from vision. Injury to a hemisphere may cause sensory deficits, depriving the brain of proprioceptive information. Many patients with injuries to the right hemisphere also have a left hemianopia (left-sided visual loss) or left spatial inattention (neglect) and fail to see or be aware of images that come from the left side of visual space. Because these patients with left arm weakness cannot see or feel their arm, they may be unaware that their arm is weak.

To determine whether this sensory feedback hypothesis could account for anosognosia, during selective right hemisphere anaesthesia we lifted patients' weak left arm and brought their left hand to the right side of their body, head, and eyes. To make certain that they could see their own hand with their normal left hemisphere, we wrote a number on their palm and asked them to read the number. After they read the number, we asked them to tell us if their hand and arm were weak. On seeing their hand, some patients who had anosognosia became aware of their weakness. Most of them, however, continued to deny weakness. These results suggest that feedback deficits are not the only mechanism that accounts for anosognosia.

Hallucination of Movements and Anosognosia

In the previous section, I described a patient named Judy Margolin, who continued to be aware of an arm that had been amputated. This phantom limb phenomenon is thought to be caused by the persistence of a memory or representation of the arm in the brain. Judy Margolin's phantom limb did not move, but John Hughes, a postdoctoral fellow who was with us several years ago, examined a patient who felt that his paralyzed limb could move. The feeling that you can move a paralyzed or nonexistent arm is called *phantom movement*. John's patient suffered a right hemisphere stroke that caused a left hemiplegia. To determine whether this man had anosognosia for this left-sided weakness, we asked him if he had any medical problems or disabilities. He said, "I guess you heard that my left arm and leg are weak." He was aware of his weakness and he could not be defined as having anosognosia, but he did not seem to be appropriately concerned about his weak and unusable arm. John Hughes spent many hours with this man. His examination revealed that he had mild spatial neglect, but he was aware of the left side of his body (no asomatognosia or personal neglect). John asked him how sure he was that his arm was weak. He answered that at first he did not think he was weak because, when he tried to use his left arm, he had the feeling that it was moving, but then he looked at the arm and discovered that it was not moving after all.

After speaking with this man about his phantom movements, we considered the possibility that these phantom movements might lead patients to believe that they were not weak, especially if, unlike this man, they are unable to monitor the arm's actions. John's patient learned that the movements he was experiencing were not real because he could attend to, inspect, and monitor his own body. Perhaps patients with severe unilateral spatial and personal neglect along with phantom movements may have anosognosia.

Disconnection Hypothesis of Anosognosia

The right and left hemispheres are joined primarily by the corpus callosum, which allows them to communicate with each other. The corpus callosum may be injured by diseases or severe head trauma. Sometimes it is also cut by neurosurgeons who treat patients with intractable epilepsy. The result is that the two hemispheres usually have trouble communicating with each other. For example, if you blindfold a patient with a callosal disconnection, put an object in her left hand, and ask her to name it, she may be unable to do so. This is because sensory information from the left hand goes directly to the sensory cortical areas of the right hemisphere, but in almost all right-handed people it is the left hemisphere that mediates language and speech. When the corpus callosum is injured, the right hemisphere,

In *Denial of Illness*, Weinstein and Kahn describe how they repeatedly asked a woman with left-sided weakness and unawareness or denial of her weakness why she was not using her left arm if it was not weak. She finally responded by telling them that her arm was not really weak but rather "lazy." Limb laziness cannot be explained by a psychological defense mechanism, by sensory feedback deficits, or by hemispheric disconnection. Laziness is a deficit in the motor-intentional systems. Perhaps this woman remained unaware of her weakness because she was unable to activate her motor-intentional systems and did not develop an expectation of limb movement because she remained unaware of her weakness.

Although the intentional or feed-forward hypothesis can explain anosognosia of weakness in some patients, other mechanisms like psychological denial, impaired feedback, impaired body image, and disconnection may also play a role in this disorder.

UNAWARENESS OF BLINDNESS

Another example of a deficit in self-awareness is anosognosia of blindness. One of the best examples of a patient with this disorder I've ever encountered was Basil Antony, a 67-year-old retired accountant, who was brought to the hospital by his wife because she thought he was confused. Although he had a history of adult-onset diabetes and high blood pressure, Mr. Anthony was doing well until the day before admission, when he had trouble finding his way around the house and appeared to have problems finding items such as his toothbrush and silverware. His family thought that his vision had worsened. Before this episode his memory had been excellent, but the day before he came to the hospital, he forgot conversations that he had had with family members and often repeated himself.

When I first examined Mr. Anthony on June 1, 1978, I asked him if he was having any problems seeing and he said, "No, my vision is fine. I need glasses to read, but otherwise my vision is good." When I asked him about his memory he said, "It is not as good as it used to be." He had no other complaints. I asked him if he knew the date. He said, "I am not sure. I did not look at the newspaper today." I told him to do the best he could. He told me, "I think it is about the eighth day of the month." I then asked, "What month and year is it now?" He said, "I am not sure. I do not keep up with those kinds of things, but I think it is about March and the year is about 1970." I then told him, "Please repeat these three words: *daisy, lamp, mirror.*" He repeated the words exactly as I said them. I then asked him to remember these words. When I asked him to count backward from 100 by sevens, he performed this test accurately and rapidly. I then asked him, "Can you remember the three words I asked you to remember?" He said, "No, I can't. I guess I really do have a problem with my memory." When I tested his reading, he was unable to read even large print, such as newspaper headlines. He was able to write a good sentence, but he had trouble finding the pen and paper with which to write and had to grope around on the surface of the table until he found these items. After watching him search for the pen and paper, I said, "It looks like you are having problems with your vision." He looked at me and answered, "I don't have my glasses." His wife, who was in the room with me, said, "Dear, you only use your glasses for reading." He said, "No, I also use them for writing." She looked in her pocketbook while saying, "I think I brought his glasses. Here they are, dear." She held out her hand to give him the glasses, but he had trouble finding them until his hand accidently hit hers. He then took the glasses out of her hand and put them on. I said to him, "Now that you have your glasses on, I want you to try and read the items on this eye chart." I held the eye chart in front of him. He asked, "Should I start on the top and read down?" I answered, "Yes." He then started saying the letters: *E, G, T, B, L, S, K.* He said each of these letters with so much conviction that although the eye chart I was showing him had numbers rather than letters, I looked at the chart to make certain I had not taken the wrong one. I considered confronting him about his confabulations but realized that neither he nor I had anything to gain. Because brain damage even in the absence of blindness may interfere with reading, I held up objects and asked him to name them. When I help up my glasses and asked him, "What object is this?" he replied, "That is a pen." When I then held up my pen and asked, "Can you name this object?" he said, "It is your watch." Some brain lesions can impair reading as well as object and face recognition, so I said, "If you see that I am holding up my hand, please point to it." Randomly I either held up my hand or did not, but in all the trials he pointed. Finally, to see if he could even detect light, I said to him, "I am going to hold a flashlight in front of your face and shine it into your eyes. Please tell me when the light goes on and off." Although he said, "Now it's on" or "Now it's off," he was often incorrect. All these visual tests indicated that he was blind.

We obtained an MRI scan of his brain that showed damage to both the right and left occipital lobes. This is the region where visual information comes to the cerebral cortex. Neurologists call this condition *cortical blindness* or *Anton's syndrome* for the neurologist who first described the disorder, including the denial of blindness. Mr. Antony had also suffered damage to the medial part of both temporal lobes, an area important for memory. This syndrome is most often caused by a blood clot that lodges in the basilar artery. This artery carries blood to both sides of the posterior portion of the brain.

The reason Mr. Antony and many other patients with cortical blindness deny their blindness is unknown. We could not attribute his condition to psychological denial because although he denied being blind, he did not deny having a memory problem. While examining Mr. Antony, I observed some behavior that allowed me to develop a hypothesis to account for his unawareness of blindness. To see if he could describe a scene, I said, "Mr. Antony, I am going to walk you over to the window, and when we get there I want you to tell me what you see outside." This window overlooked a hospital courtyard where there were chairs and tables with metal umbrellas. Since smoking was prohibited in the hospital, several patients were in the courtyard smoking and talking. I guided him over to the window and placed his hands on the window sill. After appearing to look outside for a few seconds he said, "Well there is a fenced yard that has a red and white swing set with two swings and a slide at the end. There is a grill and a white dog house." As Mr. Antony was describing what he saw, his wife looked surprised. Because of where she was sitting she could not see out of the window, so I assumed that she thought he was actually seeing these things. However, before I had a chance to explain, she said, "My husband just described our backyard. We put that swing set up for our grandchildren."

To help explain what I think may have been happening with Mr. Antony, I would like you to do a little experiment. Try answering these questions: Where is the date printed on a penny? Which way is Lincoln facing, right or left? How many printed capital letters are made entirely of straight lines? If you tried to answer these questions, you probably stopped reading or looked away from the page. You may have even closed your eyes. To answer such questions, people use visual imagery. When attempting to use visual imagery, most people cannot simultaneously process visual input fully. This suggests that both the analysis of visual input and the use of visual imagery employ the same area of the cerebral cortex. When this area is being used for one of these functions, it cannot also be used for the other functions. Our visual system may be organized in a manner similar to our home entertainment complex. We have the equivalent of a television (TV), a video camera, and a video cassette recorder (VCR). The VCR has a tape with our visual life experiences loaded on it. The camera is connected to both the TV and the VCR. The VCR is also hooked up to the TV. If the images from the camera and VCR came on the screen together, it would be difficult to see the images from either system. A properly designed system, therefore, should have cutoff switches. In humans, vision is similar to the camera and imagery is similar to the VCR. Because the VCR and camera both use the same TV screen, when one of these comes on the other one must go off. In the interest of survival, vision (the camera) should take priority over imagery (the VCR). Perhaps people close their eyes when they are attempting to use imagery because, when processing visual input, they have problems displaying their visual memories. When people's visual systems are impaired (the camera is broken), it is possible that they can no longer inhibit the visual memory systems from activating and displaying visual images. As a result, these patients see images from their visual memories. For reasons that remain unclear, patients like Mr. Antony think that these images (pictures on the TV screen) are coming from vision (camera) rather than from their visual memories (VCR).

UNAWARENESS OF APHASIA

Although there are many other forms of anosognosia, the last one I will discuss is unawareness of aphasia. Patients who are unaware of their language-speech disorders often have dramatic behavioral disorders. Analysis of these disorders may allow us to better understand self-awareness.

Shortly after moving to Gainesville from Boston, I was asked to see George Beck, a patient at the Gainesville Veterans Administration hospital with aphasia. I was wearing my white jacket, and as soon as I entered the neurology ward, Mr. Beck walked over to me. He looked at my pockets and then started speaking to me, but his speech was comprised almost completely of neologisms, or nonsense words. In the "Speech" section of Chapter 2 we discussed this type of aphasia, which was named after the neurologist who first described it, Carl Wernicke. Because these patients speak in meaningless jargon, the condition has also been called *jargon aphasia*. I tried to explain to Mr. Beck that I did not understand his speech, but his comprehension of speech was also impaired and he could not understand me. Whatever he was trying to tell me must have been important to him, because it was apparent from his speech prosody that he was very angry about something. In frustration he grabbed the lapels of my coat and started shaking my coat as he spoke. Gently but firmly, I took his hand off my coat and then made a gesture for him to be quiet. I also gestured for him to calm down. He seemed to understand these gestures, stopped speaking, and calmed down. Then I led him back to his room and to his bed. After he sat down on the bed, I went to the nurses' station and asked them about Mr. Beck, but they didn't know why he was so upset. One of the nurses suggested that, like many of the patients who smoked, he wanted a cigarette.

Although Mr. Beck had a severe speech impairment, I could tell from his actions that he was unaware of the problem. In the "Speech" section of Chapter 2, I described how Wernicke's aphasia is caused by a lesion in the part of the brain where memories of how words sound are stored. A person does not need these word sound memories to have thoughts, but without them, thoughts and needs cannot be expressed verbally so that other people can understand. When a normal person is speaking and makes a speech error, such as an incorrect sound, the speaker usually hears the mispronounced word and is able to correct the error because her or his brain contains memories or representations of how this word should sound. Because this patient with Wernicke's aphasia had lost the memory of how words sound, he not only had difficulty understanding people who spoke to him but also was unaware that his own speech was incomprehensible.

I went back to Mr. Beck's room and pantomined smoking. He smiled and nodded his head. I shook my head and showed him a picture of a nicotine patch. I had the resident physician who was looking after him prescribe a nicotine patch and an antidepressant to help him stop smoking. I also asked our speech pathologist, Dr. Leslie Gonzalez-Rothi, to teach him Amerind, a gestural language.

A loss of word sound representations is not the only cause of anosognosia of abnormal speech. Several years ago, two of our postdoctoral fellows, Lynn Maher and Jeff Shuren, told me about a patient they were evaluating who made frequent speech errors by substituting incorrect speech sounds for the sounds of certain words. For example, when asked to name objects, he called a pencil a *bencil* and my watch band a *wabsh bam*. Unlike Mr. Beck, the patient with Wernicke's aphasia who was unaware he spoke jargon, this man's comprehension of speech was good, and we could not ascribe his unawareness of his speech errors to a loss of word sound representations. To learn if he could detect errors when other people made them, we produced speech sound errors similar to those he made and asked him to indicate when we made these errors. He had no problem performing this task. This made us wonder if his unawares of speech errors was some form of psychological denial, so we taped his speech and then played it back to him. He not only was able to detect almost all of the errors he had made, but was amazed at having been unaware of these errors when he spoke. Psychological denial was obviously not the explanation. Why, then, was he unaware of his errors when he spoke?

A soldier may not detect his wounds until the battle is over. In Chapter 4, I discussed the proposition that the brain has a limited capacity to process stimuli. Patients with aphasia, such as this man, may have great difficulty expressing themselves, and their attempts to speak are often like a battle. We thought that perhaps this man was unaware of his errors because he was using all of his attentional capacity to speak and had no capacity to monitor his own speech. To test this hypothesis, we had him attempt to detect speech errors that we made purposely while he was also speaking. Unlike normal people, he was unable to do so. When normal people speak they also make errors, but these errors are infrequent. Sometimes we do not recognize such errors. Perhaps when we speak rather than attending to speech output, we are attending to our thoughts.

SUMMARY

One way to understand the brain mechanisms of self-awareness is to study patients who have lost self-awareness. In the clinic we see two disorders of self awareness: not knowing that a part of the body belongs to oneself, called *asomatognosia*, and not being aware of a disability, called *anosognosia*. One theory of anosognosia (i.e., not knowing that ones' own left arm is paralyzed) and asomatognosia (i.e., not believing that ones' left arm belongs to oneself) suggests that there is a deficit of feedback caused by either sensory deficits or inattention. Altering feedback to create awareness, however, helps only a small percentage of people with these disorders, suggesting that while feedback is important for self-awareness, other factors are also important. Another hypothesis suggests that the brain contains a representation or memory of the body, and in these conditions this representation is destroyed. Support for this representational, or body scheme, hypothesis of asomatognosia comes from the observation that patients who have a limb removed still experience the limb as being present. This observation suggests that even in the absence of feedback from a limb, the person experiences the presence of this limb because her body image is still whole. The presence of sensory representations in some patients may cause an inability to recognize a disability. Patients with blindness may deny their blindness because they see images. However, these images are coming from their memory rather than through their eyes.

The lost of a part of the body schema (asomatognosia) may also explain anosognosia for weakness. A person who has lost the representation of his left arm will be unaware that this arm belongs to him. If he does not own the arm that is not working, he may not believe that he has arm weakness. Although many patients who are unaware of their weakness also have asomatognosia, not all patients with anosognosia have asomatognosia. A loss of representations may also account for other forms of unawareness. Patients with a variety of other disorders, such as aphasic speech, may be unaware of their deficits because they have lost the monitor that contains the memories of how words should sound.

Studies of patients with injury to the corpus callosum, which connects the right and left hemispheres, suggest that the language-dominant left hemisphere may be unaware of information, intentions, or actions mediated by the right hemisphere. While in some

patients hemispheric disconnection may help explain verbal unawareness, even when the left hemisphere is able to see the left arm,
there may be still be unawareness of weakness.

A person becomes aware of a deficit when there is a mismatch
between her expectation and performance. Some patients do not
try to move and thus never develop expectations. Their disorder is
one of initiation or intention.

On the basis of these studies of asomatognosia and anosognosia,
we conclude that self-awareness is a multicomponent process. To
develop self-awareness, one must monitor oneself. This process requires both sensory feedback and a monitor. This monitor, which
contains representations or memories, must receive not only sensory
feedback but also intentions. Whereas the intentional feed-forward
system sets the monitor's expectations, the feedback system provides
the monitor with data.

Selected Readings

Critchley, M. (1969) *The parietal lobes,* Hafner, New York.

Damasio, A.R., (1999) *The feeling of what happens,* Harcourt, Brace
and Company, New York.

Feinberg, T.E., (1997) Anosognosia and confabulation. In *Behavioral
neurology and neuropsychology.* McGraw-Hill, New York, pp. 369–
380.

Heilman, K.M., Barrett, A.M., Adair, J.C. (1998) Possible mechanisms of anosognosia: a defect in self-awareness. *Phil. Trans. R.
Soc. Lond.* (Biological Science Series) 353:1903–1909.

Prigatano, G., Schacter, D. (Eds.). (1991) *Awareness of defect after brain
injury,* Oxford University Press, New York.

Weinstein, E.A., Kahn, R.C, (1955) *Denial of illness,* Charles C. Thomas, Springfield, Ill.

CHAPTER

6

MEMORY

One of the brain's major functions is to store information. The storage of information is called *memory*. Over the past 100 years, we have learned that there are least four different types of memory and that these memories are mediated by different brain systems. *Working memory* is a temporary memory store. If you are using a pay phone and do not have the telephone number of the person you want to call, you might call information. When the operator tells you the seven-digit number, you might rehearse the number until you find the coins for the phone and dial the number. Several minutes after you have finished the call, there is a good possibility that you will have forgotten this phone number because you stored the information only in working memory. In contrast, if I ask you what you had for dinner last night, you would probably recall that you had steak with fries. You would not have been rehearsing "steak and fries" since dinner time, so the information was placed in a more permanent store. This form of memory is called *declarative* or *episodic memory*. Declarative memories may be verbal (e.g., recalling names) or nonverbal (e.g., recalling faces) and may be old (remote) or new (recent). The loss of declarative memories is called *amnesia*. With declarative memories you recall "what, where, and when," but with *procedural memories* you remember "how." For example, remembering how to ride a bike is a procedural memory. Lastly, throughout life you have acquired knowledge. For example, you know the names of objects (nouns) and the words for actions (verbs). This store of knowledge is called *semantic memory*.

In this chapter we will discuss these four types of memory and the brain mechanisms that are important in storing them. Because we know most about declarative memories and the loss of these memories (amnesia), much of this chapter will be about amnesia, but we will start with a discussion of working memory.

WORKING MEMORY

After the operator gives you the telephone number and while you are looking for coins for the phone, if someone asks you when your call will be finished and you respond, there is a good possibility that you will have forgotten the number. The word *rehearse* comes from two morphemes (*re* = again and *hear*). During rehearsal one repeatedly repeats and rehears. When you were distracted, you may have stopped rehearsing and forgotten the number.

In order to rehearse, you must be able to repeat words and sentences to yourself. About 30 years ago, I noticed that many language-impaired or aphasic patients who could follow simple commands such as "Please point to the light" or "Please point to the door," could not follow more complex commands such as "Before pointing to the light, please point to the door." In order to understand a complex sentence, persons must continually repeat it to themselves until they comprehend all of its elements. Many patients with aphasia have impaired repetition, which interferes with verbal working memory.

If a person is asked to repeat numbers, and these numbers are presented at a rate of one number per second, the average person will be able to recall seven numbers (e.g., 5, 6, 3, 7, 9, 2, 4). If asked to repeat these numbers in reverse order, the average person will be able to recall only about five numbers (e.g., 4, 2, 9, 7, 3) because reversing the numbers requires more working memory. When we studied the working memory of aphasic patients who had poor repetition, we found that they could only repeat two or three numbers forward. To understand the complex command "Before pointing to the light, point to the door," one must temporarily store at least four pieces of information: *point, light, door*, and *order* (*door* before *light*). In some aphasic patients, poor comprehension of complex commands is probably related to their inability to maintain four pieces of information in working memory.

Patients with injured frontal lobes often have deficits of their working memory. Some investigators believe that the frontal lobes store working memory, but frontal lobe injuries make patients easy to distract. Because they are easily distracted, they have trouble rehearsing and perform poorly on tasks that require working memory.

DECLARATIVE MEMORY

Declarative memory is important for "knowing that." Facts, lists, and dates are all examples of declarative memory. Some neuropsychologists and neurologists equate declarative memory deficits with amnesia, but to many laypersons and media reporters, amnesia is forgetting who you are. Several times a year, emergency room staff see patients who are in all respects normal but who cannot recall their name, their past, or where they are. Patients with severe declarative memory deficits, including those with Alzheimer's disease, are almost always able to recall their name. In the absence of other neurological deficits, patients who cannot remember their own identity have psychological or functional problems rather than neurological disorders.

One of the most striking examples of a declarative memory deficit, or true amnesia, is Korsakoff's disease. When I was a neurology resident, I had a patient with this disorder. Sean Fabrec was found by the police at 6:00 A.M. on Washington Street in Boston. He appeared to be sleeping on the sidewalk. The police tried to wake him to tell him to move, but they had trouble arousing him and had him brought to the emergency room at Boston City Hospital. When I examined him there, he remained difficult to arouse. His clothing was dirty, his hair was matted, and he smelled as if he had not showered in years. He also had a rash that suggested scabies, and his matted hair was full of lice. There are hundreds of diseases that can cause people to become comatose. Immediate treatment of some of these diseases can save lives. Thus, after checking vital signs, such as pulse, respirations, temperature, and blood pressure, we often automatically treat patients for two conditions: hypoglycemia and Wernicke's encephalopathy, which is caused by the inability of alcoholics to absorb vitamin B_1, or thiamine. Immediately after Mr. Fabrec was brought to the emergency room, we placed an intravenous line (IV) and gave him thiamine and sugar (glucose) through the IV. Most patients who are brought in by ambulance and look like Mr. Fabrec have alcohol addiction. Drinking excessive alcohol prevents the body from absorbing thiamine. Without this vitamin, the neurons in the brain cannot absorb glucose, the main source of energy for the brain. While I was putting the IV into his arm, another neurology resident was drawing blood from his other arm so that we could check his blood glucose level and determine if there were other chemical or metabolic conditions that might be causing his coma. Shortly after receiving the thiamine and glucose, however, Mr. Fabrec became alert. We were then able to examine him in more detail, and we found that he could not move his eyes to either the right or the left, a sign often associated with Wernicke's encephalopathy. That Mr. Fabrec became alert after thiamine treatment and had paralysis of eye movements helped us make the diagnosis of thiamine deficiency with Wernicke's encephalopathy.

We planned to admit Mr. Fabrec to our neurology inpatient service so that we could treat him with thiamine for several days, but before this happened, the nurses bathed him, deloused him, treated him for scabies, and put him in a clean, new gown. There are many things that I like about working with the poor in city hospitals. Perhaps the most important one is that in these hospitals, patients like Mr Fabrec, who suffer from alcohol or drug addiction, are not treated as though these disorders are signs of moral weakness. Instead, these patients are treated for their disease, and addiction is certainly a frequent and disabling disease. In the future, I hope we learn that addicts are not criminals and that taking drugs is not a crime but rather a sign of a treatable disease.

Mr Fabrec was admitted on a Friday evening, but I did not have a chance to speak with him further because we did not get all the patients with emergency admissions under control until Saturday afternoon. In addition, I was scheduled to be off duty that weekend. Since Mr. Fabrec was doing well, I let the team that was on call for the weekend look after him.

On Monday morning, I made rounds with the two medical students who were assigned to our service for the month. One of them, Mike C., had Mr. Fabrec for a patient. Over the weekend, Mike, had obtained the patient's history and examined him physically, so I asked him to present his findings to our group of medical students, interns, and residents. He replied, "Mr. Fabrec is a 52-year-old Caucasian man who was doing well and was in good health. One night he was walking home after having dinner with some friends when he was robbed and mugged. After he gave the robbers all his money, they hit him over the head and left him on the street. His review of systems is negative, except that his feet feel as if they are burning. His social history reveals that he has smoked about one pack of cigarettes per day since he was a teenager. He is a social drinker. He had 2 years of college education before going into the service. He is currently a salesman at Discount Furniture in Mattapan. On examination, I found that his vital signs were normal and there were no abnormalities on his general physical examination. His neurological examination was also totally normal." I asked, "Mike, what do you think caused his coma?" He replied, "Well, I did not have a chance to look over the ER notes, but I guess head trauma." "Mike, can I show you some important physical signs that you may have missed? Look at the palms of his hands. Do they look unusual for a man?" Mike looked at Mr. Farbrec's hands and said, "They look okay to me." One of the other medical students said, "They look kind of red." I said, "Good observation. This redness is called *palmar erythema,* and you can see this in women who are taking estrogen or who are pregnant." I then asked Mr. Fabrec if Mike could feel his chest, and he nodded consent. After doing so, Mike told the group, "Yes he has breast tissue." I explained to the students that even men make some estrogen but that normally the liver is important in degrading it. Patients with liver disease cannot degrade estrogen, and increased levels of this hormone have feminizing effects. I asked, "Mike, what are the most common causes of hepatic dysfunction?" He replied, "Alcohol and viral hepatitis." Using a cool piece of metal, I demonstrated to Mike, and the other students, that Mr. Fabrec had reduced sensation in his feet, but when I rubbed his feet he complained of a burning sensation. Alcohol and poor nutrition can injure peripheral nerves, and the reduced sensation with burning may be signs of an alcoholic neuropathy. A neuropathy can also involve a decrease in tendon jerks. For example, normally when you hit the Achilles tendon, at the back of the ankle, with a rubber hammer, the foot jerks, just as the leg jerks when you hit the tendon under the kneecap. These reflexes are called *deep tendon reflexes*. Mr. Fabrec's foot did not jerk down when I hit his Achilles tendon, indicating that he had lost this reflex. I asked the medical students what this meant. Mike said that Mr. Fabrec had a sensory neuropathy (the nerves carrying messages from the foot and leg to the spinal cord and brain were working improperly). I then asked Mike, if this neuropathy might be related to his liver disease. He replied, "I guess he was drinking more alcohol than he told me."

Although Mr. Fabrec had spent the previous night in the hospital, I asked him what he had done that night. He said, "Doc, I worked in the furniture store until late, and then I took the train home and I was mugged on the MTA by a bunch of kids." When I looked at Mike, he was shaking his head in disbelief. I asked him the date. He did not know the day, the day of the week, the month, or even the year. It was 1969, and he thought it was 1958. I asked him who was president of the United States, and he answered, "Truman." Then I said, "Mr. Fabrec I want you to remember these three words: *daisy, lamp*, and *mirror*. Could you repeat those words back for me?" He said, "*Daisy, lamp*, and *mirror*." I said, "Good. Keep trying to remember the words because in 3 minutes I will ask you to recall these three words. Now, in the meantime, I would like you to subtract 7 from 100 and then continue to subtract by sevens." Mr. Fabrec was very good at arithmetic and made no errors. When he got to the number 65, I interrupted and asked him if he could recall the three words I had asked him to remember. He said, "I think so. *"MTA, Truman, kids."*

Mr. Fabrec was revealing an inability to develop new memories, a condition called *anterograde amnesia*. To learn whether he also had trouble remembering previously learned material, I asked him to name the last five presidents. His answered, "The only presidents I can remember now are Truman and Roosevelt." He did not name Johnson, Kennedy, or Eisenhower. Kennedy was one of Boston's favorite sons, and people from Boston do not easily forget his name.

When I asked him who Kennedy was, he replied, "He is our senator." Thus, in addition to being unable to store new memories, he was unable to recall some old memories. The inability to recall old memories is called *retrograde amnesia*. The finding that patients such as Mr. Fabrec can recall older memories better than recent memories is called *Ribot's rule*. No one has provided a full explanation for Ribot's rule, but some cognitive neuroscientists think that old memories are more strongly consolidated than recent ones. It is the strength of functional connections between neurons that allows our brains to store information, and old memories may be stored by neural connections that are more robust than those that store recent memories.

I asked Mike to call Discount Furniture in Mattapan to see if Mr. Fabrec was currently working there. When Mike returned he said, "I spoke with the owner of the store, who said that Mr. Fabrec used to work there but has not worked there for about 10 years. I asked the store owner how, after all these years, he could remember Mr. Fabrec so well. The owner said that Mr. Fabrec was his brother-in-law. He also said that Mr. Fabrec was a good salesman, but when he started to hit the bottle he did not show up at the store for days, so finally he had to let him go. Until we called, he had not seen or heard from him for several years."

Mike asked, "Why do you think he lied to me? Do you think it was to save face?" I said, "I don't think that he told you the truth, but I don't think he lied either. Have you ever heard the expression that the difference between a lie and a mistake is intent? When someone lies there is an intent to deceive, but when one makes a mistake, there is no such intent. In the clinic, this type of mistake is called *confabulation*. No one knows why some people with memory disorders confabulate, but some people have suggested, as you have, that patients with memory loss confabulate to fill memory gaps and avoid embarrassment. One of the best predictors of who will confabulate, however, is not the severity of memory loss but the part of the brain that is damaged, suggesting that confabulation is not a voluntary compensatory strategy but, like amnesia, results from brain damage. Often the memory episodes that patients confabulate are partially true, but as Mr. Fabrec demonstrated, their time tagging is often incorrect."

I asked Mike, "What part or parts of the brain, when injured, can cause severe amnesia?" Mike replied, "In the late nineteenth, century the Russian physician S.S. Korsakoff was the first person to describe this memory disorder in alcoholics. Then, in the early part of the twentieth century, neuropathologists thought that the critical lesion was in structures called the *mammillary bodies.*"

The mammillary bodies are so named because they resemble breasts hanging from the base of the brain (Fig. 6–1). In some people, alcohol prevents the absorption of thiamine. The drop in the thiamine level can cause hemorrhage into the mammillary bodies. The mammillary bodies are part of the hypothalamus, which exerts central control over visceral organs through the autonomic (without voluntary control) nervous system or by changing the concentrations of certain hormones in the blood. The hypothalamus changes hormone levels by sending messages to the pituitary, or master gland. For example, if a person becomes dehydrated and the blood

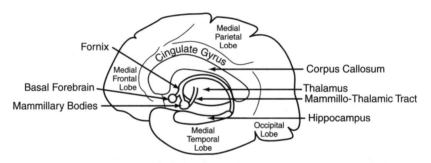

Figure 6–1. Diagram of a midsagittal section of the brain (cut through the middle of the brain and separating the brain into two halves) demonstrating the medial temporal lobe with the hippocampus. The major outflow from the hippocampus is to the fornix. The fornix carries messages to the mammillary bodies located just below the thalamus or in the hypothalamus. The mammillary bodies send messages to the thalamus by way of the mammillo-thalamic tract. From the thalamus, information is carried to the cingulate gyrus, located just above the corpus callosum. From here the messages are carried back to the hippocampus, thereby making a circuit. The hippocampus and other components of this circuit are part of the limbic system, and this circuit is named for the man who first described it, Papez. Papez thought this circuit was important for the experience of emotion, but it is now known that many parts of the circuit (the hippocampus, fornix, mammillary bodies, and mammillo-thalamic tract) are important for memory. Portions of the basal forebrain are also important for memory. The basal forebrain contains nerve cells that travel in the fornix to the hippocampus and supply it with the critical neurotransmitter acetylcholine.

becomes too thick, the hypothalamus sends a message, via the pituitary gland, to the kidneys to conserve water. However, we still do not know why, when the mammillary bodies are injured, memory loss occurs.

Maurice Victor, Raymond Adams, and George Collins studied the brains of people who had a history of severe alcohol abuse and died. They found that in patients with Korsokoff's syndrome, there was damage to both the mammillary bodies and part of the thalamus. However, patients without memory loss may have damage to the mammillary bodies but not to the thalamus. These observations suggest that mammillary body injury alone may not cause amnesia. Other investigators have studied stroke patients with injury of the thalamus or the pathway from the mammillary bodies to the thalamus and found that these patients had amnesia. Lynn Speedie and I demonstrated that people with strokes that injure the medial part of their left thalamus, have verbal memory loss, and those with strokes that injure the right part of the thalamus have visual-spatial memory loss (e.g., faces). Because Mr. Fabrec had both verbal and nonverbal memory loss, it is possible that both his right and left thalamus were damaged.

Although Mr. Fabrec was no longer drinking alcohol, and was being treated with thiamine and other vitamins, his memory never returned to normal. No member of his family agreed to take him to their home, so we placed him in a nursing home.

Damage to other parts of the brain may also cause amnesia. One of the most common causes of amnesia is damage to the temporal lobes. The patient who taught us the most about memory and the temporal lobes is H.M., an epileptic man studied extensively by Brenda Milner and her colleagues. The temporal lobes often give rise to the abnormal electrical currents that cause epileptic seizures. Many patients with seizures can be treated with drugs that control these abnormal currents, but some cannot be treated successfully and their seizures occur so often that they cannot lead a normal life. Because these seizures originate in a specific area of the brain, neurosurgeons sometimes remove this area. Although removal of part of the temporal lobe, called *temporal lobectomy*, is a standard procedure that has afforded many patients relief from disabling epilepsy, when neurosurgeons started performing it, H.M., one of their first patients, suffered a severe side effect. Before surgery, his brain waves were recorded by EEG to demonstrate where the seizures started in his brain. Two epileptic foci were found, one in the left temporal lobe and the other in the right. Therefore, the surgeons removed the anterior portion of H.M.'s right and left temporal lobes, including the hippocampus (Fig. 6–1).

After H.M. recovered from surgery, his epilepsy was better controlled but he become severely amnesic. Although H.M.'s intelligence was unchanged and he retained many of the memories he had formed before the operation, he was unable to learn and retain new information. Brenda Milner, who worked in the Montreal Neurological Institute, and Sue Corkin, who now works at MIT, studied his memory for years, but he never recognized them and they had to introduce themselves each time they met him. Nor could he recall conversations he had a few minutes after they were over. He did not remember current events and even had trouble recalling the day, month, or year.

After H.M.'s terrible experience, neurologists and neurosurgeons recognized that they could operate only on patients whose seizures originated in one temporal lobe. When the anterior portion of one temporal lobe is removed, patients still have memory deficits, but usually these are so mild that they do not prevent the patient from living an independent and productive life. When the left temporal lobe is removed, verbal memory is impaired; removal of the right temporal lobe leads to impaired spatial memory. In one neuropsychological test, patients are shown pictures of people's faces they have not previously seen and are asked to remember them. After being distracted, the patients are shown a card with these same faces mixed together with foils (faces they have not been shown previously). Patients with right temporal lobectomy, but not those with left, have difficulty identifying the faces they have previously seen. In contrast, when patients with left temporal lobectomy are given a list of words or a story to remember, after distraction they have difficulty remembering the words or the story, but when given the face memory test they perform normally.

In the 1950s, when performing temporal lobectomies, surgeons removed the entire anterior portion of the temporal lobe. This region contained *neocortex* (new cortex in evolutionary terms), including portions of both the auditory and visual association cortices. The medial inferior portion of the temporal lobe also contains evolutionarily primitive cortex that is part of the limbic system (Fig. 6–1). Subsequent studies revealed that it was not the removal of neocortex that caused the memory loss, but rather the removal of this more ancient cortex. The part of the limbic system that most researchers now think is important for memory is called the *hippocampus.*

Blows to the head, strokes, a severe drop in the level of oxygen (*hypoxia*) or sugar (*hypoglycemia*) in the blood, viruses such as *herpes* (cold sore) virus, and even strokes may injure the hippocampus and cause amnesia. Alzheimer's disease is probably the most common cause of amnesia from damage to the hippocampal formation.

The hippocampus is connected to the mammillary bodies by a structure called the *fornix* (Fig. 6–1). The hippocampus-fornix and mammillary bodies are part of a circuit (Fig. 6–1) that was first thought to play a role in emotional experiences but is now known to be important for memory. Up to about 25 years ago, it was unclear whether damage to the fornix produces a memory deficit in humans. Then George Sypert, a neurosurgeon at the University of Florida, saw a patient named Flora Pape, who was referred from a neurologist in Jacksonville because she was having progressive memory loss. Her evaluation revealed that she had a tumor involving both the right and left fornices. Dr. Sypert surgically removed the tumor. Unfortunately, to remove the tumor completely, he had to remove both fornices. Mrs. Pape had lived in eastern Kentucky all her life until she and her husband moved to Jacksonville, about 2 years before surgery. She had two sons in their twenties, both of whom had remained in Kentucky. When she was discharged from the hospital, her husband drove her from Gainesville to their home in Jacksonville. After leaving Gainesville, her husband noticed that she was looking out the window and saying, "Oh, my!" He asked what was troubling her and she said, "What happened to the mountains?" He asked, "What mountains?" She replied, "You know, the mountains." He said, "There are no mountains here." She replied, "No mountains in Kentucky. We must be in the western part of the state. What are we doing here?" Mr. Pape had been told by Dr. Sypert that the surgery might make her memory worse, but he was still surprised. "Dear, we are not in Kentucky. We are in Florida." She asked, "Why are we in Florida?" He told her that they had moved to Jacksonville about 2 years earlier. She said, "Moved to Jacksonville? Why?" He told her that the company had asked him to transfer. She asked, "Where are we going now?" "Back to Jacksonville from Gainesville. You had some surgery on your brain. It was a tumor.

The doctors think they got it all out. You are having some memory problems, but the surgeons hope it will improve with time." Then she asked, "Who is watching the boys?" "No one." he replied. "They are grown and live in Kentucky." "What do you mean, grown? They are still teenagers." "No, they are not. They are in their twenties. They are coming down this weekend to see you." She stopped asking questions for a few minutes and looked out of the car window. Then she turned to her husband and asked, "Where are all the mountains?"

George Sypert arranged for Mrs. Pape to see me. I tested her intelligence and memory. It appeared that she had retrograde amnesia that went back for several years. To determine if she had anterograde amnesia, I read her a story and then asked her to repeat it. Immediately after I read the story she was able to recall some of the details, but not as many as she should have remembered. After about 30 minutes, I asked her to again tell me as much about the story as she could and she asked, "What story?" I told her that the story was about a ship that sank, but she was still unable to recall any parts of it. Although she had profound anterograde and retrograde amnesia, her IQ was normal. Unfortunately, there are no drugs that can cure or even significantly improve amnesia. I spent several hours with Mrs. Pape and her husband talking about strategies they could use to help deal with this memory loss, including using memory notebooks, labeling items around the house, and using written reminders such as "Please record all phone messages on this pad."

After neural information leaves the hippocampus, travels via the fornix to the mammillary bodies, and then travels from the mammillary bodies to the thalamus, it returns to the hippocampus via the cingulate gyrus (Fig. 6–1). At the back of the cingulate gyrus, behind the back end of the corpus callosum (called the *splenium*), is an area called the *retrosplenial cortex*. Ed Valenstein and other people from our laboratory reported a man who had a hemorrhage that destroyed the retrosplenial cortex. He had profound amnesia and was similar clinically to H.M., Mr. Fabrec, and Mrs. Pape. Studies of these important patients suggest that damage to this hippocampus–fornix–mammillary bodies–thalamus–retrosplenial circuit can cause amnesia. Studies in monkeys by Mort Mishkin, Larry Squire, and Stuart Zola have confirmed that this circuit is important in forming declarative memories.

One nerve activates another by emitting a chemical called a *neurotransmitter*. In the hippocampus the most important neurotransmitter is acetylcholine. Some drugs may interfere with the action of acetylcholine. When I was in medical school, I used one of these drugs when I was on the obstetrics service. We had to learn how to deliver babies and spent 4 weeks on this service. First, we observed residents delivering one or two babies; then they observed as we performed deliveries. These residents were following the old medical school educational dictum "See one, do one." The first woman I took care of was a girl of 16. This was her first baby, and she seemed to be in a lot pain during labor. I spoke with the resident physician in charge of her case about giving her something to reduce the pain, but he disagreed. Each time she had a labor contraction, she screamed in pain. She kept asking for a painkiller, and I went back to the resident physician. He answered, "If we give her a painkiller it will affect her child, who will be born sleepy, and this will reduce the child's chances of doing well. I will order some scopolamine for her."

Before our clinical rotations, we had taken a required pharmacology course and learned that scopolamine is an anticholinergic medication. I knew that scopolamine had several uses, but I had never learned that it reduces pain. The resident offered this clarification: "It will not kill her pain, but she will not remember that she had it."

When I returned to the girl's room, she was ready to deliver. In the delivery room, the nurse gave her an injection of scopolamine. Her labor pains continued. When she was about to give birth, the resident made a small incision at the mouth of the vagina (episiotomy) to allow the infant's head to emerge without tearing the vagina. Before cutting, he gave her a local anesthetic, but this did not stop the labor pains. The resident then allowed me to deliver the baby as the girl screamed. The infant girl was healthy, breathed immediately, and started to cry. After we cut the umbilical cord, the nurse and the pediatric resident took the baby, cleaned it, and then gave it to the mother to hold. When she saw her beautiful baby and held it in her arms, this young mother finally stopped screaming and started crying. While I cleaned her and sewed up the vaginal wound, I told her that everything looked good and she had a beautiful baby.

Shortly after the delivery she fell asleep. When I made rounds with the resident the next morning, we asked her if she was glad that the delivery was over. She said, "You know, I can hardly remember anything about the birth."

I never expressed my misgivings to the resident, but I thought that there must have been a safe means of reducing her suffering. Today scopolamine is rarely used in the delivery room, and there are several methods for reducing pain without making the baby sleepy. However, I was intrigued that scopolamine could prevent a woman from recalling one of the most important events of her life.

At the base of the brain is an area called the *basal forebrain*, which is responsible for supplying the hippocampus with acetylcholine. The basal forebrain is connected with the hippocampus by the fornix (Fig. 6–1). Injury to the basal forebrain can destroy the cholinergic neurons that send acetylcholine to the hippocampus. Several years ago, we took care of a high school principal from Daytona who had a severe memory loss from injury to the basal forebrain. This man was healthy except for having had epileptic seizures for more than 20 years. He was taking the anticonvulsant Dilantin but was still having about one seizure every 3 months. These seizures did not interfere with his life, except that they prevented him from driving. When CT scans became available, he was given several scans to make certain that a brain tumor was not causing these seizures, but no tumor was found. When MRI became available, his doctor ordered a scan to see if there was any abnormality the CT scan had missed. It revealed a small tumor in his basal forebrain. His physician sent him to a surgeon, who decided to remove the tumor. The rationale for removal was never clear to me. If this tumor was causing his seizures, it had probably been present for so long that it must have been benign. The surgeon may have thought that if the tumor was removed the seizures would diminish, but it was never clear that the tumor was the cause of the seizures. In any case, the surgeon called the operation a success because the patient survived, did not bleed, and did not become infected. When this patient's family visited him in the hospital, however, he could not even recall why he had the surgery. When we examined him, he had profound anterograde amnesia and some retrograde amnesia. The surgeon hoped that this memory loss would be transient, but it did not improve.

We thought that perhaps when the surgeon removed the tumor, he injured the cells that supply acetylcholine to the hippocampus. To test this hypothesis, we performed functional imaging (single photon emission computed tomography, [SPECT]), which uses a radioisotope. The radioisotope is injected into the blood and a machine measures the radiation in the brain. The higher the radiation level in an area of the brain, the greater the blood flow to that area. When a portion of the brain becomes active, blood flow to this area increases. Thus, by measuring the radiation level, we can ascertain which areas of the brain are active. When we measured the amount of radioisotope going to this man's hippocampus we found it to be abnormally low, suggesting that the hippocampus was not active. This decrease in activity was probably related to the surgery in the basal forebrain, which had destroyed the cells that supply the hippocampus with acetylcholine. This patient was similar to the girl in the delivery room who was given scopolamine, the drug that blocks acetylcholine. But whereas her amnesia was temporary, this man's was permanent.

Several months after he was discharged from the hospital the patient tried to return to his job as a principal, but was unsuccessful because of his poor memory. He also developed many interpersonal problems. We were planning to treat his memory loss by giving him a medicine that increases the level of acetylcholine, but before we could do so he had a massive heart attack and died.

In patients with Alzheimer's disease, amnesia is usually one of the first symptoms. This disease damages both the hippocampus and the basal forebrain, which supplies acetylcholine to the hippocampus. Based on this knowledge, physicians hoped that if they could increase the level of acetylcholine in these patients' brains, their memory would improve. Several drugs are now available that do increase the level of brain acetylcholine, but these drugs do not fully restore memory because increasing acetylcholine does not restore cells in the hippocampal system.

PROCEDURAL MEMORY

Whereas the declarative memory system stores "who, what, and where" information, the procedural memory system stores "how" knowledge. Patients who have deficits of declarative memory, or amnesia, may have intact procedural memory. H.M., the patient who developed severe amnesia after both of his temporal lobes were removed, was given a motor learning task called *rotor pursuit*. As part of this task he was given a metal wand to hold in his right hand. On a table in front of him was an apparatus that looked like an old phonograph turntable. On top of the turntable was a little metal disk about the size of a quarter. H.M. was told to try to keep the wand on the little metal disk while the turntable rotated. When learning a new motor skill such as rotor pursuit, the more normal people practice, the more skilled they become at keeping the wand on the metal target. Each day H.M. was brought into the laboratory to practice rotor pursuit. Each time this happened, he never recognized the examiner or knew the goal of the task. So, each day the examiner had to introduce herself and give him instructions on how to use the rotor pursuit apparatus. Although H.M. could not recall the task's instructions, he did improve with practice. H.M. demonstrated that procedural (how) and declarative (when, who, what) memories are dissociable and that the hippocampus–fornix–mammillary body system (also called the *Papez circuit*) is important for declarative but not procedural memories.

Dan Jacobs and other people from our laboratory also used rotor pursuit to test patients with Alzheimer's disease. These patients, like H.M., had amnesia. All the patients also had a semantic memory deficit (discussed below), and some had a working memory deficit. Despite impaired declarative, working, and semantic memory, when using the rotor pursuit these patients' performance improved with practice, demonstrating that they had normal procedural memory. In contrast, Nelson Butters and his coworkers showed that patients with Parkinson's disease who had normal declarative, semantic, and working memory were impaired on motor learning. Patients with Parkinson's disease have a reduced level of the neurotransmitter dopamine. This neurotransmitter impairs function of the basal ganglia–motor cortex circuits (see Fig. 9–3), and it is these circuits that must be important in developing procedural memories.

SEMANTIC MEMORY

Semantic memories are stored knowledge about the world. For example, the names of objects and actions are semantic memories. Semantic memory deficits such as impaired naming are discussed in other chapters and will be considered only briefly here.

The most common cause of impaired semantic memory is Alzheimer's disease. Patients with this disease, for example, may be unable to name objects correctly (*anomia*), recognize objects that have been named, or even know the purpose of certain objects (*object agnosia*). They may forget the procedures of addition and multiplication and be unable to calculate (*acalculia*), fail to recognize and name body parts (e.g., *finger agnosia*), and be unable to recall where to find items (*topographic disorientation*). In addition, patients with Alzheimer's disease have impaired declarative memory (amnesia). John Hodges described another degenerative disorder, which he calls *semantic dementia*, characterized by a relatively isolated semantic memory deficit. Semantic memories appear to be stored in the parietal and temporal lobes. The left lobe stores verbal-language semantic memories and the right lobe nonverbal visual-spatial semantic memories. In Alzheimer's disease and semantic dementia, these regions degenerate.

Further evidence for the dissociation of declarative and semantic memories comes from studying the vocabularies of people who have a long history of amnesia. The vocabulary tests used for this purpose were designed to ascertain if these amnestic patients knew words that had been invented after they were injured. Each year, many new words are invented. Two recent additions are *e-mail* and *Internet*. In spite of having severe amnesia these people learned new vocabulary words, providing further support for the independence of declarative and semantic memories. Patients with Parkinson's disease who have impaired procedural memory may have normal semantic and declarative memories. Further, as mentioned earlier, patients with Alzheimer's disease who have impaired semantic memory may have good procedural memory. Thus, observations of patients with Alzheimer's disease, Parkinson's disease, and Korsokoff's syndrome reveal that the working, procedural, semantic, and declarative memory systems are functionally and anatomically independent (i.e., modular systems). Verbal working memory depends on the dorsolateral frontal lobes and the left perisylvian speech areas. Declarative memory is mediated by a hippocampal–fornix–mammillary body–thalamic–posterior cingulate (retrosplenial) circuit, the Papez circuit. Procedural memory is dependent upon basal ganglia–cortical loops, and semantic memories are stored in the temporal and parietal cortex.

SUMMARY

Human beings have four different types of memory: working, declarative, semantic, and procedural. The systems that mediate these
different forms of memory are functionally and anatomically independent (i.e., modular systems). Working memory is a temporary
store. To keep information there, the person must actively rehearse
the information that is being stored and prevent distraction. The
left frontal lobe is important in verbal working memory and the
right frontal lobe in spatial working memory. Declarative memory
stores, "what, where, and when" information. Declarative memories
may be verbal (e.g., recalling names) or nonverbal (e.g., recalling
faces) and old (remote) or new (recent). The areas that are important for storing declarative memories are located primarily in the
Papez circuit (hippocampus–fornix–mammillary bodies–thalamus–
cingulate gyrus–retrospenial cortex–hippocampus). This memory
system is illustrated in Figure 6–1. The hippocampus, which has extensive connections with the cerebral cortex, requires acetylcholine
to store and retrieve memories. The cell bodies of the neurons that
send acetylcholine to the hippocampus are located in the basal forebrain, and injury to this area causes an amnesia similar to that associated with injury to portions of the Papez circuit. Knowledge, or
semantic memories, is stored in the temporal and parietal regions
of the cerebral cortex. Verbal declarative and semantic memories
are stored in the left hemisphere and visual spatial memories are
stored in the right hemisphere. Procedural memories are "how"
memories. Although the network that encodes procedural memories
has not been fully elucidated, basal ganglia interactions with the
cortex appear to be important.

Suggested Readings

Baddeley, A.D. (1986) *Working memory*, Oxford University Press,
    Oxford.
Bauer, R.M., Tobias, B. Valenstein, E. (1993) Amnestic disorders. In
    Clinical neuropsychology. (Ed.) Heilmen, K.M., and Valenstein, E.,
    Oxford University Press, New York, pp. 523–602.
Boller, F., Grafman, J., Cermak, L.J. (Eds.). (2000) *Handbook of neu-
    ropsychology: Memory and its disorders*, 2nd ed. Elsevier,
    Amsterdam.

McCarthy, R.A, Warrington, E.K. (1990) Short term memory, auto-biographical memory, and material-specific memory. In *Cognitive neuropsychology*, Academic Press, New York, pp. 275–342.

Schacter, D.L. (2001) *The seven sins of memory: How the mind forgets and remembers*, Houghton Mifflin, New York.

Squire, L.R. (1987) *Memory and brain*, Oxford University Press, New York.

the major link between the cortices of the left and right hemispheres. Hemorrhages like Mrs. Calla's can either cause death or leave the patient with brain damage. The hemorrhage causes vessels to go into spasm, and in this state they cannot deliver a normal amount of blood to the portions of the brain they serve. Mrs. Calla's hemorrhage was located between the two hemispheres on top of the corpus callosum, suggesting that the artery that normally provides blood to the corpus callosum was the one that hemorrhaged and went into spasm, damaging the callosum.

To test functionally the possibility that the corpus callosum was injured and could not transfer information between the hemispheres, we blindfolded Mrs. Calla and gave her objects to feel and name. Although she flawlessly named objects that were placed in her right hand, she could not name anything placed in her left hand. She was successful at naming objects placed in her right hand because the sensory impulses go from this hand to the left hemisphere, which mediates language. When Mrs. Calla held objects in her left hand, however, the sensory information went to her right hemisphere, which is without language. For her to name the objects in her left hand, this sensory information had to be sent to the left hemisphere from the right by way of the corpus callosum. This patient's ability to name objects in her right but not her left hand provided functional evidence that she had sustained damage to the major interhemispheric connection, the corpus callosum. Our clinical impressions were confirmed when an MRI scan showed damage to the corpus callosum.

Damage to the corpus callosum, therefore, can cause an interhemispheric disconnection. Perhaps Mrs. Calla could not carry out verbal commands with her left arm and hand because the command to pantomime had to be decoded by the left hemisphere, and this decoded information could not gain access to the right hemisphere's motor system, which controls the left hand. To test this possibility, we asked her to watch us pantomime an action (e.g., using a pair of scissors) and then to copy our pantomime. Unlike pantomiming to a verbal command, imitating does not require language. Mrs. Calla could imitate almost perfectly with her right hand but not with her left hand. We then gave her actual tools and objects to use with her right and left hands. Again, she performed well with her right hand but very poorly with her left. Because imitating and using actual tools and objects do not require language, her inability to perform these tasks could not be explained by a disconnection between the left hemisphere's language system and the right hemisphere's motor system. Some other information stored in the left hemisphere had been disconnected from the right hemisphere.

In the early twentieth century, Hugo Liepmann, who had been a student of Carl Wernicke, observed a similar case and suggested that in addition to language, the left hemisphere of right-handed people stores what he termed *movement formulas*. These formulas contain the temporal and spatial knowledge of how to perform learned, skilled movements. Because these memories, or representations, of how to perform skilled movements are stored in the left hemisphere, destruction of the corpus callosum would disconnect them from the motor system in the right hemisphere. This is what accounted for Mrs. Calla's inability to pantomime correctly to command, imitate gestures, and use tools correctly with her left hand.

Left Hemisphere Lesions

In the clinic we often see right-handed patients who have had strokes of the left hemisphere. Most of these patients come to our clinic because they have speech problems. Often they also have weakness of the right arm. When we test their ability to perform skilled movements with their left arm, they often demonstrate apraxia and pantomime poorly the use of tools and objects (transitive gestures). They also have difficulty imitating the examiner pantomiming transitive gestures and using actual tools.

Until about 30 years ago, many neurologists thought that this inability to pantomime correctly was related to language deficits. They thought that the left hemisphere was important for using symbols, and whereas aphasia is the inability to use speech symbols, apraxia is the inability to use gestural symbols. Viewing apraxia and aphasia as disorders of symbol use, they called these disorders *asymbolia*. There are, however, two major problems with this explanation of apraxia. First, patients with apraxia are impaired even when they are using actual tools. Second, in the clinic, we see patients with aphasia who do not have apraxia and patients with apraxia who do not have aphasia. If two signs or symptoms are dissociable, then there cannot be one cause or mechanism such as asymbolia for both.

Norman Geschwind attempted to explain the apraxia caused by left hemisphere lesions by using a disconnection model in which one part of the brain is disconnected from another. When someone is given a verbal command such as "Show me how you would use a pair of scissors to cut a piece of paper in half," this command first goes to the primary auditory area in the left hemisphere (Fig. 7–2). After it is analyzed by the primary auditory area, this information goes to Wernicke's area, located in the posterior portion of the left temporal lobe, which is critical for speech comprehension. According to Geschwind's model, after the command is decoded in Wernicke's area, it must go to the premotor area on the left side in order to reach the primary motor cortex. The premotor cortex is located immediately in front of the primary motor cortex, which is located just in front of the central sulcus that separates the frontal and parietal lobes. If the right hand is to be used, this information

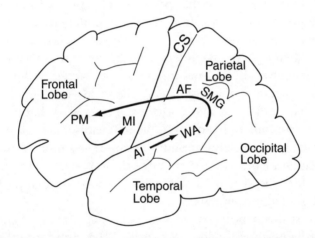

Figure 7–2. Diagram of Geschwind's model of praxis (performing a skilled, learned movement to command) drawn on a diagram of the left hemisphere demonstrating the motor cortex (M1), which is located directly in front of the central sulcus (CS). The CS divides the frontal lobe from the parietal lobe. Auditory information comes to the primary auditory cortex (A1) and then proceeds to Wernicke's area (WA), which is critical for comprehending the verbal command. After the message is decoded, it is carried to the frontal lobes to an area just in front of the motor cortex called the *premotor cortex* (PM). This information is carried by a white matter pathway called the *arcuate fasiculus* (AF), which connects Wernicke's area to the premotor cortex. This pathway travels under the supramarginal gyrus (SMG). From the PM the information goes to the motor cortex (M1) which sends the message to the spinal cord. The spinal cord has nerve cells that send messages to the muscle through peripheral nerves.

then goes to the left hemisphere's motor cortex and the command is implemented. If the left hand is to be used, however, the information must travel by way of the corpus callosum to the right premotor cortex and then to the motor cortex of the right hemisphere. From Wernicke's area in the left hemisphere, information about the command reaches the premotor cortex via an arc-shaped pathway called the *arcuate fasiculus*, located below the cerebral cortex. When patients have apraxia from left hemisphere lesions, the area most commonly injured is the supramarginal gyrus (Figs. 7–2). The arcuate fasiculus runs under the supramarginal gyrus, and Geschwind thought that when this pathway was damaged, the information about the command could not move from Wernicke's area to the premotor areas.

Unfortunately, Geschwind's disconnection model cannot account for the observation that patients with apraxia from left hemisphere lesions also are impaired when they imitate transitive gestures or use actual tools and objects. When the left hemisphere is injured, the right hemisphere has intact sensory systems, and the cortical areas that analyze this sensory input also have access to the premotor and motor areas of the right hemisphere. My colleagues (Ed Valenstein and Leslie Gonzales-Roth) and I suggested that perhaps injury to the supramarginal gyrus of the left hemisphere causes apraxia of both the left and right forelimbs because the supramarginal gyrus is the region of the brain that stores the representations, or memories, of how the arm and hand should be moved when performing learned, skilled movements.

To test this hypothesis, we examined patients who had apraxia from left hemisphere lesions. We divided the group into those with posterior lesions that included the supramarginal gyrus and those with anterior lesions that had not injured the supramarginal gyrus. If our hypothesis was correct, apraxic patients with posterior lesions should also be impaired in discriminating between correctly and incorrectly performed pantomimes. They should be impaired because they have lost the memories, or representations, of the spatial and temporal characteristics of these learned, skilled movements. In contrast, patients who are apraxic from more anterior lesions should have intact movement representations and should be able to make these discriminations correctly. We showed the patients movies of an actor pantomiming skilled acts. Sometimes the actor performed the movements correctly, and sometimes he made errors. Whereas

the patients with anterior lesions could determine which pantomimes were correct and which were incorrect, the patients with posterior lesions could not. These results support the hypothesis that in
right-handed people the representations of learned, skilled movements are stored in the supramarginal gyrus of the left hemisphere
and that when these movement memories are destroyed, patients
cannot perform skilled movements correctly with either hand or
recognize when someone else makes errors while performing skilled
acts.

We often see aphasic patients in our clinic who also have
apraxia, but most of them are unaware of their deficits of motor
control. Many of these patients have right-sided weakness (hemipa-
resis) and attribute their left-hand clumsiness to the use of their
nonpreferred hand. Many patients who do not have right-sided
weakness are also unaware that they have lost the ability to perform
skilled movements with their right hand. This is a form of *anosognosia*
(*a* = without; *noso* = disease or disability; *gnosia* = knowledge), or
unawareness of a disability. If a person makes any type of performance error, the only way he or she can recognize the error is to
know what is correct and to be able to compare his or her own
performance to a mental image of a correct performance. Many
patients with apraxia have lost the representations of learned, skilled
movements, and perhaps they are unaware that they are impaired
because they no longer know what is correct and what is incorrect.

According to the model of motor control we have discussed
(Fig. 7–3), the left inferior parietal region contains the spatial and
temporal memories of how to perform learned, skilled movements,
and the corticospinal system activates the nerves that make the muscles in the arm move. For example, if you want to slice a piece of
bread from a loaf, the parietal lobe stores the knowledge that the
shoulder must move alternatively forward and backward at the same
time that the elbow is alternatively flexed (bent) and extended
(straightened). The knowledge stored in the left inferior parietal
lobe is a representation of a movement (the temporal and spatial
characteristics of a skill) but not of a motor program. For example,
a movement representation may tell us how a movement looks but
not which muscles we have to use to make this movement. A motor
program provides instructions as to which nerves have to be activated in order to make the muscles in the arm contract so that it
performs a slicing motion. The premotor cortex receives the nec-

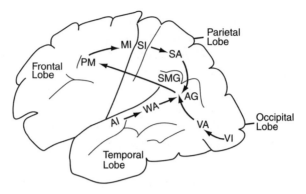

Figure 7–3. Model of the praxis system. The memories of how to move through space and the speed with which one must move are stored in the region of the supramarginal gyri (SMG) or angular gyri (AG), which together comprise the inferior parietal lobe. These movement memories, or representations, can be activated by verbal commands through auditory cortex (A1) and Wernicke's area (WA) or visual stimuli through visual cortex (V1 and VA) or tactile stimuli through somatosensory cortex (S1 and SA). These spatial and temporal movement memories activate neurons in the premotor cortex (PM), which converts this spatial-temporal information into a motor code or program that, in turn, activates the motor cortex (M1). The motor cortex has nerves that go down to the spinal cord, which sends peripheral nerves to the muscles that implement the programmed movements.

essary information from the parietal lobe and forwards it to the motor cortex. Patients with lesions of the premotor cortex are unable to carry out skilled acts but are aware of their errors and can discriminate well-performed from poorly performed movements. It appears that the premotor cortex is important for developing motor programs based on the spatial and temporal information it receives from the parietal lobe. The premotor cortex uses motor programs to activate the appropriate portions of the motor cortex that send messages to the spinal cord, the peripheral nerves, and finally the muscles that implement skilled movements.

PRAXIS AND HANDEDNESS

About 90% of people prefer to use their right hand to perform skilled acts (right-handers). The other 10% either prefer to use their left hand (left-handers) or can use either hand equally well. Although hand preference is one of the most striking asymmetries found in people, the explanation for it is still not entirely clear.

In many cultures, left-handedness has negative social implications. Our scientific word for left-hand preference is *sinistral.* This word comes from the Latin root *sinister,* which means "evil." Because left-handedness was thought to be evil, there was a social stigma about using the left hand. Today in American schools and homes, it is rare for left-handed children to be forced to write and perform other skilled movements with their right hand, but several generations ago, training left-handers to use their right hand, especially when writing, was common practice. One theory of hand preference is the learning theory, which suggests that social pressures and learning rather than biological factors determine hand preference. This theory is not supported by the fact that social pressures against using the left hand are now rare in our society, but the prevalence of left-hand preference remains about the same.

In 1863 Paul Broca described eight patients with left hemisphere injury. All were right-handed, and all had aphasia. Based on these observations, Broca suggested that in most right-handed people it is the left hemisphere that mediates language and speech. Subsequent investigations confirmed this hypothesis. This led to the view that hand preference is related to language laterality. If a person hears a command to perform a skilled action, the command is decoded by the speech-language areas in the left hemisphere. The nerve cells that control movements of the right hand are also located in the left hemisphere, so using the right hand is more efficient than using the left hand, which would require information to be transferred from the left to the right hemisphere.

One method of learning about the relationship between hemispheric language dominance (language laterality) and hand preference is to study patients while one of their hemispheres is not working. To learn which hemisphere mediates language in patients who may undergo neurosurgery, each hemisphere is put to sleep by injecting short-acting barbiturates into the arteries that feed blood into one hemisphere and then the other. In a group of left-handed patients, this test revealed that 70% used their left hemisphere to mediate language. Another 15% used the right hemisphere to mediate language, and the remaining 15% used both hemispheres.

These observations demonstrate a dissociation between hand preference and language laterality, indicating that language laterality is
not the major factor that determines hand preference.

In 1973 I saw a retired farmer, Ralph Corry, who had grown up
in southern Georgia. He was visiting his son, who lived in Gainesville,
when he had a sudden onset of left-sided weakness. In the emergency room, he told me that when this weakness started his son was
not home. He wanted to call an ambulance to take him to the hospital and also wanted to leave a note for his son telling him what
had happened and where he was going, but he found that he could
not write with his right hand. Since boyhood he had always written
with his right hand, and it was his left, not his right hand, that was
weak. He could not understand why he could not now write with his
right hand. The examination did demonstrate that his left arm was
weak and that most of this weakness was in his hand. His speech and
language were entirely normal. When I tested his writing by asking
him to write a sentence about the weather, he gave the impression
that he had never learned to write because he did not know how to
form letters. He was able to read normally and could spell aloud the
words he could not write. He had never learned to type, but I provided a typewriter and asked him to type a sentence about the
weather. By using the forefinger of his right hand, he could type out
words that he could not write in longhand.

There are two major causes of *agraphia* (inability to write correctly): *aphasic (language-spelling) agraphia* and *apraxic (motor)
agraphia*. Because Mr. Corry could type but not write, it appeared
that he had apraxic agraphia. His language was intact, but he had
either lost the knowledge of how to form letters or could not perform the skilled movements needed to do so.

When I asked Mr. Corry to pantomime skilled acts such as using
scissors or a screwdriver with his right hand, his performance was
very poor. He made severe spatial errors and seemed to be apraxic.
I asked him if he was right-or left-handed. His mother had told him
that he was a natural southpaw, but at school he was taught to write
with his right hand. When he told me he was a southpaw, I asked
him if he played baseball. It turned out that he had been a pitcher
and played baseball in the minor leagues but never made the majors.
I asked him if he pitched with his left hand, and he said "Yes."

This left-handed man had lost the ability to write with his right hand because even when he learned how to write with his right hand, he continued to store movement representations in his right hemisphere. Unlike Mr. Corry, natural right-handers store this information in their left hemisphere. We thought that Mr. Corry had had a stroke that had damaged much of his right hemisphere, including the movement memories, or representations, that are important for knowing how to form letters and how to perform other skilled movements. His injured right hemisphere could not provide movement information to the left hemisphere, which controlled his right hand.

Hugo Liepmann, the neurologist who initiated the study of apraxia at the beginning of the twentieth century, thought that it was these lateralized movement representations that were responsible for hand preference. He thought that people with right-hand preference have their movement representations stored in the left hemisphere and those with left-hand preference in the right hemisphere. If these representations are lateralized to one hemisphere, then when one performs a skilled task such as writing, control over the hand on the opposite side is direct but control of the hand on the same side is indirect. That is, the right hemisphere's motor neurons project directly to the part of the spinal cord that controls the muscles in the left hand, and the left hemisphere's motor neurons project to the part of the spinal cord that controls the muscles in the right hand. If a person with left-hand preference, such as Mr. Corry, wants to write with the right hand, the information about the necessary movements, stored in the right hemisphere, must first be transferred from the right to the left hemisphere by way of the corpus callosum. Although people can learn to use this transcallosal route, as Mr. Corry did, this route is indirect and less efficient. According to Liepmann, it is the laterality of these movement representations, rather than language lateralization, that determines hand preference.

Although Liepmann thought that hemispheric laterality of movement representations determines hand preference, we do not think it is the only factor. Along with Steve Rapcsak, we have seen two patients who had right-hand preference, and were never forced to switch from left-to right-hand preference, but developed apraxia after suffering right hemisphere damage. One of these patients was also aphasic, suggesting that his right hemisphere also mediated language. Although it is not clear why this man preferred to use his right hand to perform skilled acts, there are other factors that may influence hand preference.

People have many physical asymmetries. In most but not all people, for instance, the heart is on the left side and the liver is on the right side. Most men have one testicle that is larger than the other, and most women have one breast that is larger than the other. There are also asymmetries of the hands and arms. When using one hand to perform a task, a person may select the hand and arm that are stronger or more deft and can move more rapidly or precisely. Several studies have demonstrated that we often prefer the hand that is more deft. Although muscle mass may be an important factor in determining strength, one cannot predict strength based on muscle size alone. The means by which the nerves activate a muscle also help determine its strength. Unfortunately, little is known about what determines asymmetries of strength, but we do know that the motor nerves that originate in the cortex and run to the spinal cord are important for deftness (e.g., speed and precision). Since the time of the phrenologist Franz Gall, many brain scientists have accepted the postulate that bigger is better. In our laboratory, Anne Foundas found that the part of the motor cortex that controls the hand is larger on the left side than on the right side in people who prefer to use their right hand. Although asymmetries of strength and deftness may influence handedness, some people prefer to use their right hand even though they are stronger and more deft with their left hand and vice versa. These observations suggest that asymmetries of strength and deftness cannot be the only factors that determine hand preference. In addition, researchers have demonstrated that the brain changes with practice. For example, if one practices a skill that requires speed or precision, the cortical region that controls the hand on the opposite side may grow larger. This observation suggests that some asymmetries such as deftness may be a function of experience and this experience is a product of the lateralization of the movement, discussed above.

In addition to language, praxis, deftness, and strength, there are other behavioral asymmetries that may influence hand preference, including attentional symmetries. For example, Mieke Verfaellie and others in our laboratory have demonstrated that when a right-handed person prepares to use the right hand, he or she attends to both the left and right halves of body-centered space, but when this person prepares to use the left hand, he or she attends primarily to the left half of space. In many activities in which one has to interact with environmental stimuli, having a wider attention window provides an advantage. Overall, it appear that the hand one favors is probably determined by a host of factors, the major ones being the laterality of motor (praxis) programs and deftness.

MECHANICAL KNOWLEDGE

The best way to determine if patients have lost their movement representations is to ask them to pantomime a transitive movement such as pretending to use a pair of scissors to cut a piece of paper in half. Many patients who are unable to perform this pantomime command correctly, or even to imitate correctly a movement the examiner has just made, may be able to improve their performance when given an actual pair of scissors and a piece of paper. Based on observations such as these, several neurologists have thought that apraxia is a disorder seen only in the laboratory. Studies in our laboratory have demonstrated that using actual tools and objects does indeed improve performance. Using the actual object restricts the number of possible movements, and the object itself provides strong cues. Still, patients often make timing and spatial errors. To learn whether patients are impaired when performing routine activities of daily living, we decided to videotape patients who had had strokes when they were using tools and implements.

One morning after making rounds, I was returning to my office when I passed by a bathroom with an open door. Cindy Ochipa was videotaping a patient, George Lewis, who was about to brush his teeth. Mr. Lewis was left-handed and had suffered a stroke in the posterior portion of his right hemisphere. He picked up the toothpaste in his left hand and the toothbrush in his right hand. After briefly looking at each hand, he started brushing his teeth with the tube of toothpaste in his left hand.

I had never seen anything like this. I thought that Mr. Lewis had a problem recognizing objects (*object agnosia*), but most agnosias affect only one sensory modality, such as vision. Unlike patients with agnosia, he not only looked at the objects in his hand but also felt them and still misused them. I asked Cindy if I could interrupt her videotaping to test him for agnosia. After introducing myself, I showed Mr. Lewis the toothbrush and asked him to name it. He said, "Looks like a toothbrush." I then showed him the tube of tooth-paste and asked him to name this object. He said, "A tube of Colgate toothpaste." Then I asked Cindy to bring him back to his bed after he had brushed his teeth. I collected a few more tools and objects from my office and went to his room. He was able to name any object I showed him without difficulty, except for mispronouncing the word *stethoscope*. Patients with agnosia cannot name tools and objects that they do not recognize. Thus, Mr. Lewis did not have visual agnosia.

We asked the ward nurse if Mr. Lewis was having trouble with other activities involving the use of tools, such as eating. She said, "No, he seems to be just fine." We returned just before lunch to videotape him eating. After the food came and the tray was placed on his bed stand, the nurse helped him prepare his food by cutting the meat and putting sugar in his tea. She then took away all the utensils except his fork. Superb nurses such as this woman know intuitively the type of assistance that patients require, and she was providing this help almost automatically. We interrupted Mr. Lewis's lunch before he started eating and put back the spoon, the knife, and a toothbrush as well to see if he would use the correct utensils. Instead of using the teaspoon to stir his iced tea, he used a knife, and rather than stir it, he kept the knife stable and rotated the glass with his other hand. Along with meat on the main dish, there was creamed corn. Using the toothbrush, Mr. Lewis tried to pick up the corn, but it kept falling off. Eventually, he moved his index finger down the toothbrush to the part that contained the bristles so that he could trap some of the corn between the bristles and his finger. Using this finger chopstick method, he was able to place some of the corn in his mouth. His be-havior suggested that this man had lost his knowledge of tools and the purpose for which they are used. He no longer understood the mechanical advantage provided by each tool.

After a few minutes, we did what the nurse had done previously and made sure that the only tool Mr. Lewis had was a fork. After his food was prepared, he was able to eat his lunch using the fork alone. After finishing, he had some creamed corn on his chin. He took a slice of white bread and used it to pat his lips and chin as if it were a napkin.

If Mr. Lewis did not know the intended use of tools, he would also have difficulty answering questions about them. I asked him, "If you want to make a small hole through a piece of wood, what tool would you use?" He answered, "To cut wood, I would use scissors." From his responses to this and similar questions, it appeared that he had indeed lost his knowledge of the purpose of tools.

Perhaps just as one gains knowledge about a variety of topics, such as the different types of animals, food, clothing, and transportation, one also gains mechanical knowledge. The observation that Mr. Lewis had no trouble answering questions about these other forms of knowledge suggests that mechanical knowledge is stored separately.

We use tools because they provide us with a mechanical advantage which allows us to perform tasks we could not perform using our hands alone. Based on our observations of Mr. Lewis, we tested several forms of tool knowledge, or what we call *action semantics*, in groups of right-handed patients who had had strokes of either their right or left hemisphere. We wanted to determine if they knew what action is associated with each tool. For example, did they know that a twisting movement is used with screwdrivers? We wanted to find out if they knew which tool was associated with a particular object. If shown a nail, for example, could they select a hammer rather than a knife, ice pick, scissors, or hand saw? We also wanted to learn if patients knew the mechanical advantages that tools can afford. To answer this question, we tested patients with an alternative tools test. For example, in one trial we placed a board with a nail that was partially driven into it in front of these patients. Between the patients and the board we placed five tools: a hammer, a plier, a screwdriver, a knife, and a hand saw. We asked each patient to point to the tool he or she would use to complete the task. If the patient selected the hammer, we took it away and then asked again which tool would be best to finish the task. In this trial the correct answer was the plier because is hard and has a heavy head.

The most difficult mechanical task is to develop tools to solve a mechanical problem. We had our patients attempt to retrieve a red wooden block from a Plexiglas tube. In the first half of the trial, they could use their hands to withdraw the block. If they succeeded, we gave them a similar puzzle, but this time they could not use their hands. Instead, they had to make a tool from the material we supplied to lift the block out of the tube. For example, in one pair of puzzles, the edges of the block were so close to the tube that the patient could not grasp the block. However, on top of the block was an eyelet, and the block could be removed by pulling on it. In the second part of the puzzle, the tube was too small to allow insertion of a hand. Next to the puzzle was a piece of aluminum wire. To retrieve the block, the patient had to bend the end of the wire, make a hook, and use it to lift the block out of the tube.

Many of the right-handed patients with left hemisphere injury had trouble with these tests of mechanical knowledge. Right-handed patients with right hemisphere injury rarely had trouble. Many of the patients who had lost mechanical knowledge also had trouble pantomiming skilled acts, indicating that the temporal–spatial, or praxis, knowledge of how to use tools is often stored in the same hemisphere as mechanical knowledge important for tasks, such as tool selection. However, some patients who had lost mechanical knowledge could pantomime normally, and some patients who could not pantomime correctly had normal mechanical knowledge. This dissociation indicates that although mechanical knowledge and movement knowledge are often stored in the same hemisphere, these systems are independent.

SUMMARY

To perform skilled acts (praxis), people need movement programs and mechanical knowledge. Movement, or praxis, programs are the instructions given to the nerves that control the limbs. These programs instruct the muscles about what joint or joints to move, in which direction, at what time, with what speed, and with how much force. Studies of patients with hemispheric injuries provide evidence for left hemisphere praxis dominance in right-handed people and right hemisphere praxis dominance in left-handed people. Studies of right-handed patients with focal hemisphere damage suggest that praxis memories are stored in the left inferior parietal lobe. The premotor cortex, located directly in front of the motor cortex, receives the movement information from the parietal lobe. The premotor cortex is important for developing motor programs based on the spatial and temporal information it receives from the parietal lobe and sending these programs to the primary motor cortex. This praxis system is summarized diagrammatically in Figure 7–3.

We use tools because they provide us with a mechanical advantage, which allows us to perform tasks we could not perform using our hands alone. Studies of patients demonstrate that mechanical knowledge is stored independently of other forms of knowledge, such as movement programs and language. In right-handed people this mechanical knowledge is also stored in the left hemisphere, but it is not known where in the hemisphere these stores are located.

Selected Readings

De Ajuriaguerra, J., Tissot, R. (1969) The apraxias. In *Handbook of clinical neurology*, Vol. 4. (Ed.) Vincken, P.J., and Bruyn, G.W., North Holland, Amsterdam, pp. 48–66.

Geschwind, N. (1965) Disconnexion syndromes in animals and man. *Brain* 88:237–294, 585–644.

Heilman, K.M., Rothi, L.J.G, (1993) Apraxia. In *clinical neuropsychology*. (Ed.) Heilman, K.M., and Valenstein, E., Oxford University Press, New York, pp. 141–167.

Rothi, L.J.G., Heilman, K.M. (1997) *Apraxia: The neuropsychology of action*, Psychology Press, Hove, United Kingdom.

Roy, E.A. (Ed.). (1985) *Neuropsychological studies of apraxia*, Elsevier, Amsterdam.

CHAPTER
8

SENSORY PERCEPTION AND RECOGNITION

In order to successfully interact with the environment, people have to perceive visual, auditory, and tactile stimuli and then determine the meaning of these perceptions. The study of patients with brain injuries described in this chapter, allows us to begin to understand the means by which the brain perceives and recognizes stimuli.

VISION

Object Agnosia: Inability to Recognize Objects

The term *agnosia* (*a* = without; *gnosis* = knowledge)was first used by Sigmund Freud to describe the behavior of patients who could see and had normal visual acuity but were unable to recognize common objects. Agnosia has been reported in the visual, auditory, and tactile sensory modalities but is most common in vision.

One of the most interesting patients I have seen with the loss of visual recognition of objects, called *visual object agnosia*, was Joanne Wilson. Mrs. Wilson was one of Florida's wealthiest women. Her first symptom was an inability to recognize money, the item she treasured most because she had been brought up in poverty. Her father had left her mother and the family when Joanne was 6 years old. She had a brother who was then 3 and a sister who was 1. In school Joanne was an excellent student who unlike many of her girl friends, got straight *A*'s, in math. However, she started working in middle school and never finished high school because she had to work full time to help support her family. When Joanne was 18, her mother died and she took full responsibility for her younger siblings. She became a real estate broker and made enough money to send her brother and sister to college. In her late twenties she met an accountant, married, and had one son. During the second World War her husband was killed in France, but after the war she made a fortune selling houses.

Her son, a tax lawyer, brought Mrs. Wilson to our clinic because she was doing strange things. While shopping at Wal-Mart, she bought a new bath towel that was on sale for $3.99. According to her son, she never bought anything that was not on sale. When she went to pay at the checkout counter, she opened her purse, took out two $20 bills, and gave them to the cashier. In her purse, however, her son saw that she also had a $5 bill and a $10 bill. The cashier returned one of the $20 bills and gave her the change from the other bill. As she and her son walked outside and headed to the car, he asked her why she gave the cashier two $20's. She said that was all she had. He told her that she needed to have her eyes checked. Her reply was that she had just had them checked, and they were fine. Mrs. Wilson's son told me that his mother never made an error with money. When he noticed that she had trouble recognizing sales coupons in the newspaper, he took her to the ophthalmologist. The ophthalmologist examined her eyes and found that with her current glasses her acuity was fine. When her son asked what he thought was wrong her vision, the ophthalmologist suggested that she visit our neurocognitive clinic.

Mrs. Wilson was 70 years old and had been perfectly healthy all her life. She was taking no medicine, not even vitamins, "which are a waste of money." She had no other symptoms and even denied that she was having trouble with her vision. She was fully oriented and knew the day, month, year, and place. I gave her three words to remember (*daisy, lamp,* and *mirror*) and then asked her to subtract from 100 by sevens. She rapidly said, "93, 86, 79, 72, 65, 58, 51." When I interrupted to ask her to repeat the three words I had asked her to recall she said, "*Daisy,* which is my favorite flower, *lamp,* and *mirror.*"

I then gave Mrs. Wilson the Boston Naming Test, which involves showing the patient line drawings of 60 objects. At the beginning of the test the objects portrayed are very common, such as a bed and a tree, but at the end of the test they are much less common, such as a scroll and an abacus. When I showed Mrs. Wilson the first picture, which was a bed, she said, "I do not know what that is." I gave her a cue by making the sound of the first letter. She still could not name the bed. I then gave her a different type of cue by saying that it was something people slept on. She said, "Is it a bed?" Next, I showed her a picture of a tree and asked if she recognized it. She said, "I see some black markings on the page, but I don't know what this is." A sound cue did not help her, but when I told her that the object had leaves, she said, "Tree?" Although she was able to name one or two pictures without prompting, she had great difficulty recognizing most of the objects.

Sometimes patients with speech-language disorders (aphasia) have trouble naming because they cannot access the memories, or representations, of how words sound (*anomia*). Mrs. Wilson's problem, however, was not a language problem because she could say the name when given the definition. To determine if her defective perceptual recognition affected other sensory modalities, I asked her to close her eyes and then name the coins that I would put in her hand. She asked, "Can I keep them if I name them correctly?" I said, "Sure!" She then turned to her son and said, "I like this doctor." I put either pennies, dimes, nickels, quarters, or half dollars in her hand. She named all of them correctly, but when I asked her to open her eyes and name the coins I showed her, she could name only the pennies because of their color. With the other coins she did no better than chance. I tested her visual acuity while she was wearing her glasses, and as her ophthalmologist had said, it was normal.

To recognize an object, a person must first be able to perceive it. The occipital lobes receive visual information from the retina. When the person is shown pictures, like those on the Boston Naming

Test, specific portions of the occipital visual cortex detect lines or changes in brightness (edges) that are oriented in specific directions and positioned in specific portions of space. For the brain to derive meaning when the person sees an object, it must put these lines or edges together to form a percept of the object's shape. If these pieces are not put together and a percept of the object is not fully formed, the person will not be able to recognize it. This disorder of perception is called *apperceptive agnosia.*

Patients with apperceptive agnosia cannot recognize objects visually because they cannot form a visual percept. If a person can draw an object they cannot recognize, the problem is not apperceptive agnosia. To learn whether Mrs. Wilson was unable to recognize objects on the Boston Naming Test due to apperceptive agnosia, I asked her to copy the picture of the bed. Although she was able to copy this picture well, she still could not recognize that it was a drawing of a bed. Thus, Mrs. Wilson did not have apperceptive agnosia. However, in the clinic we do see patients who have injures to both occipital lobes and who are unable to recognize objects, describe what they are viewing, match the object they are viewing to samples versus foils, or draw these objects. These patients have apperceptive agnosia.

If patients can perceive objects, as determined by their ability to draw them or to match them to samples of the same objects, but cannot recognize objects by naming them, describing them, or demonstrating their use, they have *associative agnosia.* Associative agnosia may not be a unitary disorder. There may be two or more types. To explain this disorder, an analogy with aphasic disorders may be helpful. Recall that understanding speech requires at least three operations: auditory analysis of the incoming sounds, activation of the phonological lexicon (a memory store of previously heard words), and semantic processing to derive meaning. Sometimes we can hear words, know that they are English words, but not know their meaning. Similarly, when we see objects, we may be able to recall that we have previously seen similar objects because we have perceptual object memories, or representations, but we do not know their attributes, properties, or functions (semantic information). Thus, just as the phonological lexicon is independent of semantics, object perceptual representations may be independent of semantics. If these visual representations of objects are destroyed, patients will have one form of associative agnosia. Alternatively, if these object representations are intact but patients are unable to access semantic information about them, they will be unable to recognize or name objects even though they are able to draw these objects, a second form of associative agnosia (Fig. 8–1).

To learn which form of visual associative agnosia Mrs. Wilson had, we showed her drawings of real objects and nonobjects. On each page, but in different locations, we put a drawing of a real object and a nonobject (Fig. 8–2) and asked her to point to the real object. When presented with the first picture, she said, "I am not sure I can do this." But then she went on to perform flawlessly, always pointing to the real objects. In contrast, when we asked her to either name or describe the function of these real objects, she was able to name only 1 out of 30 real objects. Because Mrs. Wilson could name these objects when their function was described to her verbally, we knew that her verbal lexicon and her semantics were intact. Based on these tests, we concluded that Mrs. Wilson's asso-

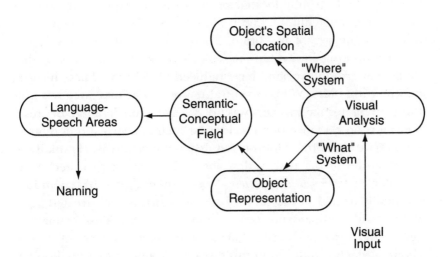

Figure 8–1. Model of the visual recognition system. When a person sees an object, after visual analysis (e.g., line position, direction, color) the visual information activates a visual object representation (percept of the shape of the object). This percept representation then accesses the conceptual–semantic field where meaning is determined. Injury to the areas of the brain that prevent visual stimuli from gaining access to visual object representations causes apperceptive agnosia. Injury that distroys these representations or prevents them from gaining access to the semantic–conceptual field causes associative agnosia.

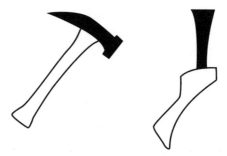

Figure 8–2. Object versus nonobject test. In this test the patient is shown a series of pages. On each page is a picture of a real object and a nonobject. The patient is told to point to the real object.

ciative agnosia was caused by a failure of object perceptual representations to access semantic representations or meaning.

To determine whether a structural disease was causing her problem, we ordered an MRI of her brain. This scan demonstrated only some cerebral atrophy located primarily in the ventral (lower) region of the left temporal and occipital lobes. We also obtained radioisotope images of her brain. These images indicate how much blood is flowing into different regions of the brain. Areas of the brain that are not working have reduced blood flow. These images indicated that Mrs. Wilson's ventral temporal occipital area was not functioning normally since it was not receiving much blood. Because there was no evidence of a focal lesion such as a stroke or a tumor, we thought that Mrs. Wilson had a degenerative disease. Frank Benson was one of the first to describe such patients; he called their disorder *posterior cortical atrophy*. Most patients with this condition eventually turned out to have Alzheimer's disease. We treated Mrs. Wilson with antioxidants (e.g., vitamin E), an anti-inflammatory agent, and Aricept (a drug that helps increase the level of acetylcholine, which is reduced in this disease). Although we were hoping to slow down the degenerative process, her disease progressed and eventually she needed full-time care.

Prosopagnosia: Inability to Recognize Familar Faces

In our first examination of Mrs. Wilson, we tested her ability to recognize faces by showing her a series of 12 pictures of famous people. These faces included former presidents, movie stars, and sport heros. She named all the faces except one (Richard Nixon) but was able to tell us that he was the president who had been forced out of the White House. Because faces are no easier to recognize than inanimate objects such as a bed, her preserved ability to recognize faces but not objects suggests that knowledge of faces is mediated by an area of the brain that is different from the areas that are important for recognizing objects.

There are patients who have *prosopagnosia* (*prosop* = face; *a* = without; *gnosis* = knowledge) and, unlike Mrs. Wilson, are unable to recognize familiar faces. Lamar Simpkins, who had graduated from the University of Florida College of Architecture 10 years before I saw him, had this problem. Lamar had a job in Orlando designing a new Lutheran church. In addition to his job, Lamar liked motorcycles, women, and beer. One day, while enjoying all three, he hit railroad tracks and crashed into a concrete power pole near Orlando. He was not wearing a crash helmet, and his head smashed into the pole. When the police and fire rescue team arrived, he was comatose and remained so when he was brought to the Orange County Medical Center. The woman who had been riding with him was released after a cut on her knee was washed and dressed. People with severe head injuries often develop blood clots under the skull (*epidural* or *subdural hematomas*) that can press on the brain and even cause death. To preserve life and brain functions, these clots must be removed immediately. After being admitted to the hospital, Lamar was sent for an emergency CT brain scan. The scan showed that he had a large blood clot in the ventral region of the right temporal and occipital lobes (Fig. 8–3). There was also a smaller blood clot in the left ventral temporal-occipital region.

The neurosurgeons were consulted, but they did not want to operate because the hematomas were not pressing severely enough on his brain to endanger his life. If they tried to remove the clots, they would have to cut through normal brain. They believed that the hematomas would resolve spontaneously. After a few hours, Lamar regained consciousness and appeared to be doing well except for a few problems, including a severe headache and some confusion. His family wanted to obtain a second opinion about removing the hematomas and had him transferred to the neurosurgical service at Shands Teaching Hospital the University of Florida. The neurosurgeons there agreed with those in Orlando. They did not want to remove the blood clots but instead decided to watch Lamar closely to make certain that his neurological status did not deteriorate.

One day when the neurosurgeons were making rounds, Lamar's

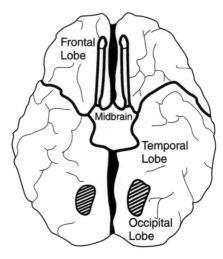

Figure 8–3. Diagram of the injuries and blood clots in the ventral portion of the occipital and temporal lobes that were found in Lamar Simpkins's brain.

sister and mother were there and asked how long they thought he would remain confused. Shortly after Lamar entered Shands Teaching Hospital, one of the neurosurgical residents had tested his memory and orientation. Many people with severe head trauma have both retrograde and anterograde amnesia. This resident found that Lamar was totally oriented. He knew the date, the day of the week, the month, and the year. He also knew the name of the hospital and the city where it was located. To test Lamar further for anterograde amnesia, the resident gave him the names of three unrelated objects to remember, and after 3 minutes he asked Lamar to recall them. Lamar was able to recall all three. Although he could not remember what had happened just before the accident, he knew what he had done at work that same day. Because of his normal performance on these memory and orientation tests, the neurosurgeons were surprised that the family thought he was confused. When people have head injuries, especially when there is bleeding into the brain, they sometimes develop epilepsy. As soon as he was admitted, Lamar was given an anticonvulsant, but on two occasions he did see colored pinwheels. These might have signaled seizure activity in his visual cortex. After a seizure, a person may be confused. At first, the neurosurgeons were concerned that perhaps Lamar had had another seizure, but one of them asked the family if this confusion had developed that day. Lamar's sister said, "No, he's had this problem since the accident. When we walk into the room, he doesn't recognize us until we tell him who we are." The neurosurgeon then asked the neurologists to see Lamar.

We first tested Lamar's mental abilities. Although he had suffered a serious head injury, his mental status was well preserved. He had no memory defects except the slight retrograde amnesia that the neurosurgeons observed. Because his major injury appeared to be located in the ventral portion of the temporal-occipital region, we decided to perform detailed testing of his visual functions. I told Lamar to look at my nose and to tell me when he saw my fingers. He could see my fingers when they were below his eye level but not when they were above it. This suggested that he was blind in the upper portion of his visual field in both eyes. This visual field defect is consistent with an injury to the lower portion of both occipital or temporal lobes. If the dorsal portion of his visual cortex had been injured in the occipital lobe, he would have had difficulty seeing below eye level. Injuries to the ventral portion of the occipital and temporal lobes may produce an object agnosia like the one Mrs. Wilson displayed. To test this possibility, we gave Lamar the Boston Naming Test. The only thing he could not name correctly was a pair of ice tongs. This demonstrated that he did not have object agnosia. Patients with ventral damage can also lose their ability to read, but Lamar had always been a good reader and was still able to read. Finally, patients with ventral temporal-occipital lesions may have difficulty recognizing faces, and this seemed to be what Lamar's sister was reporting. When we showed him 12 pictures of famous faces, he could not name or recognize any of them.

There are several reasons why a person might be unable to recognize famous faces. One is poor visual acuity, but we found that Lamar's vision was 20/20 (normal) in each eye and that he could even read small newspaper print. A second possibility is a perceptual disorder. Lamar might have been able to see parts of the face but unable to put all the parts together to construct a complete face. To test this possibility, we showed him 12 pairs of faces of people he did not know. Some were two pictures of the same person, taken from different angles with different shading, while others were pictures of two different people. Lamar performed perfectly on this test, which meant that he could perceive faces. A third possibility is that he had lost the knowledge of the identity of the famous people, but when we described these people to Lamar without showing him the pictures (e.g., "This was the president during World War II"), he was able to name all the famous people in the test.

Although we cannot be certain about the cause of prosopagnosia, we think that the brain stores visual memories of faces (facial iconic representations) of people we have previously seen and that these memories can be destroyed by brain injuries. To test this hypothesis, we asked Lamar questions about famous peoples' faces (e.g., "Was President Ford bald?"). If he had lost the memories of how these people looked, he should have been unable to answer these questions correctly. Lamar performed this test very poorly. Thus, we thought that the brain injury from his motorcycle accident had destroyed the visual memories of faces that he had previously learned.

While we were testing Lamar, a group of physicians and students of both sexes were in his room. Some wore white coats and others did not. His sister happened to enter the room then. When she approached the bed, he looked up and said, "Hi, Doc. Do you have more tests for me?" His sister smiled and said, "Lamar!" The moment he heard her voice, he said, "Sis. I'm sorry, I didn't recognize you."

After he was discharged from the hospital, Lamar came to see me every 6 months for 10 years. He never learned to recognize my face, which suggested that this injury was also preventing him from learning new faces. He also never regained the ability to recognize his family, friends, or famous people. Otherwise, his memory and thinking remained excellent.

It is not completely understood why some patients with ventral damage cannot recognize faces (prosopagnosia) but can recognize objects, whereas others cannot recognize objects (object agnosia) but can recognize faces. While most patients who have either object agnosia or prosopagnosia have lesions of both hemispheres, Lamar had a much larger lesion of the right than the left hemisphere. Some investigators have found that lesions confined to the right hemisphere can cause prosopagnosia. Todd Feinberg, together with our group, has reported a patient with object agnosia from a lesion restricted to the left ventral temporal-occipital cortex. If you have a normal person look straight ahead and then flash pictures of faces to either the left or the right side of the area where he or she is looking, the faces flashed on the left (visual field) go to the right hemisphere's occipital lobe and those flashed on the right (visual field) go to the left hemisphere's occipital lobe. Studies of normal subjects reveal that they recognize faces flashed to the left better than those flashed to the right. Furthermore, functional imaging studies of normal subjects indicate that whereas the right hemisphere is more important than the left in the recognition of faces, the left is more important than the right in the recognition of objects.

The reason for this left–right dichotomy is unknown, but it appears that the right hemisphere's approach to processing stimuli is more global and the left hemisphere's approach is more focal. Faces are very similar, and can change with aging and emotional expressions. A global approach that processes the overall facial configuration may be important for recognizing faces. By contrast, many objects have one or more critical elements that distinguish them from other objects. For example, the difference between a screwdriver and an ice pick may not be the handle or shaft but rather the distal end of the shaft. Thus, a local approach that focuses on the tip may set these two tools apart.

The biological reason that each hemisphere has a different approach to analyzing visual stimuli is not fully known, but since the time of David Hubel and Torsten Weisel's Nobel Prize-winning research on the physiology of the visual (occipital) cortex, it has been known that neurons in this area have *receptive fields*. If you look straight ahead and a light is flashed 10 degrees to the left of where you are looking, certain cells in your right visual cortex will become active. If this light is moved to different positions, these same cells may become inactive, while others begin to fire. By recording the response of these brain cells to light in different viewer-centered spatial positions in animals, maps can be drawn of the spatial zones where light causes cells to fire. The area of space where a neuron responds to a stimulus is its receptive field. It may be that neurons in the right hemisphere of humans have larger receptive fields than those in the left hemisphere. This asymmetry could give the right hemisphere an advantage in performing more global, or spatially distributed, processing while allowing the left hemisphere to perform local processing.

Spatial Disorientation

In Chapter 4 we reported that when a patient named Mrs. George was presented with pictures of complex scenes, such as a Civil War battle, she could see only one element in the scene. Mrs. George

had suffered strokes that damaged both her left and right parietal
lobes. When I first examined her, I held my index finger about 30
inches in front of her face and asked her to touch my finger with
her eyes open. Most normal people have no trouble with this test
and can touch the experimenter's index finger accurately. Mrs.
George, however, performed this task very poorly. She moved her
finger either too far or not far enough, or too much to the right or
left. When she finally touched my index finger with hers, she appeared to find my finger only by chance. Although Mrs. George had
this problem when using either hand, I also examined a patient with
a stroke of the right superior parietal lobe alone who had this same
localization difficulty, but only when she was using her left hand on
the left side of her body. This disorder in reaching a target is called
optic ataxia (*optic* = visual; *ataxia* = without order).

Leslie Ungerleider and Mortimer Mishkin observed that after
visual stimuli enter the primary visual cortex of monkeys, in the
occipital lobe, they are analyzed and processed by two visual streams.
The dorsal stream goes to the parietal lobes, and the ventral stream
goes to the ventral temporal lobes (see Fig. 4–8). The ventral stream
is important in recognizing objects or people and has been called
the *what system*; the dorsal stream is important for spatial location
and has been called the *where system*.

Patients with injury to the ventral stream have "what" recognition problems and may not be able to recognize faces or objects
(prosopagnosia and object agnosia). People with dorsal stream injuries, such as Mrs. George, have "where" problems and may have
trouble computing location. Although Mrs. George was able to recognize my finger, she had trouble knowing or computing where it
was in relation to her body. For example, when normal subjects see
a finger, using information they get from their eyes they locate the
finger and "chart," or represent, it in a three-dimensional grid that
stores the radial distance (distance from their body, or z axis), the
vertical distance (the height, or y axis), and the horizontal or right–
left position in relation to the body (the x axis). Mrs. George's parietal lesions had destroyed the portion of the brain that either com-
putes or stores this information.

Mrs. George's spatial, or "where," difficulties were not limited to
touching my finger. When a person performs a task that requires vision, the eyes move so that the critical image falls on the most sensitive
part of the retina, called the *fovea*. When Mrs. George tried to direct

strate how to use the objects correctly. Thus, callosal disconnection causes tactile anomia (a naming disorder) rather than tactile agnosia, a recognition disorder that is also called *astereognosia* (*a* = without; *stereo* = three-dimensional space; *gnosia* = knowledge).

Tactile Agnosia (Astereognosia): Inability to Recognize Objects by Touch

Failure of object recognition with preserved elemental touch sensation is most often caused by lesions involving the postcentral gyrus, the most anterior portion of the parietal lobe. Although this is the primary somatosensory cortex that receives touch sensations, this area of the brain is not needed to recognize that one is being touched. Rather, it is important when one must interpret the meaning of the tactile stimulus. Blindfolded patients with lesions of the postcentral gyrus may also have difficulty recognizing numbers or letters traced on the hand opposite their injury. This disorder is called *agraphesthesia* (*a* = without; *graph* = writing; *esthesia* = feeling. Most patients with agraphesthesia or astereognosis cannot draw what they feel and cannot match what they feel to a sample mixed with foils, suggesting that these tactile agnosias are caused by perceptual disorders (apperceptive agnosias). There have been one or two case reports, however, of patients who did not have a perceptual disorder (could match to a sample) but did not recognize objects palpated by the hand that was contralateral to a parietal lesion. As with associative agnosia in other sensory modalities, the brain injury must have dissociated the sensory percept from the semantic networks.

SUMMARY

Studies of patients with disorders of recognition suggest that the brain recognizes meaningful stimuli by using a multicomponent sequential process. Primary sensory cortices in the occipital lobes (vision), anterior parietal lobes (touch), and superior temporal lobes (audition) receive incoming sensory information and analyze it (e.g., the location and color of stimuli). This processed information is passed on to modality-specific cortical association areas that are adjacent to the primary sensory cortical areas. These sensory association areas synthesize modality-specific information and develop percepts (e.g., an image of the viewed object). In each modality-specific association area, there are representations, or memories, of percepts that have been previously experienced. The incoming sensory information activates these stored representations. These stores are also activated when a person performs activities such as drawing or using imagery. The observation that brain injury might cause a person to lose one class of percepts such as familiar faces, but not other percepts such as the forms of inanimate objects, suggests that even within a modality such as vision, different types of percepts are stored in different parts of the brain. For example, memories of familiar faces may be stored primarily in the right ventral temporal-occipital lobe, and images of inanimate objects may be stored in an analogous area in the left hemisphere. After stored percepts are activated, they normally access semantic–conceptual networks found in supramodal cortical areas such as the posterior dorsolateral temporal lobe and the inferior parietal lobe.

Selected Readings

Alexander, M.P., Albert, M.L. (1983) The anatomic basis of visual agnosia. In *Localization in neuropsychology*. (Ed.) Kertesz, A., Academic Press, New York, pp. 293–418.

Bauer, R.M. (1993) Agnosia. In *Clinical neuropsychology*. Heilman, K.M., and Valenstein, E., Oxford University Press, New York, pp. 523–602.

Benton, A., Tranel, D. (1993) Visuoperceptual, visuospatial and visuoconstructive disorders. In *Clinical neuropsychology*. (Ed.) Heilman, K.M., and Valenstein, E., Oxford University Press, New York, pp. 168–215.

Farah, M.J. (1990) *Visual agnosia: Disorders of object recognition and what they tell us about normal Vision*, MIT Press, Cambridge, Mass.

Geschwind, N. (1965) Disconnexion syndromes in animals and man. *Brain* 88:237–294, 585–644.

McCarthy, R.A., Warrington, E.K., (1990) Object recognition; face recognition. In *Cognitive neuropsychology*. Academic Press, New York, pp. 22–72.

CHAPTER

9

CONATION
AND
INTENTION

The term *conation* derives from the Latin word *conato* which means "attempt." The word, however, is defined as the initiative to act arising from within oneself. The cognitive systems (e.g., language, spatial and motor skills) provide the person with knowledge of how to operate in the environment, but they do not provide the knowledge of when to interact with it. There are three intentional, or "when," decisions that a person must make: (*1*) when to act, (*2*) when to persist at an act, and (*3*) when not to act. We will start our discussion of intentional systems by describing people who have lost their initiative.

ABULIA: LOSS OF INITIATIVE

Perhaps the first person to be described with *abulia* (*a* = without; *bulia* = will) was Phineas Gage in John Harlow's 1868 report. In the mid-nineteenth century, Gage, a hard-working foreman of a railroad crew, had an accident in which an iron tamping bar, used to place explosives, was propelled by an explosion upward into his skull. The rod entered the left cheek, went through the maxillary sinus on the left side, and impaled the frontal lobes of his brain. It then exited the top of the skull. That Gage survived such an accident was remarkable. It was also remarkable that as a result of this accident he did not become weak and was able to speak normally. He did, however, undergo a dramatic personality change. Before the accident, according to Harlow, Gage had "a well balanced mind. And was looked upon by those who knew him as a shrewd, smart business-man, very energetic and persistent in executing all his plans." After the accident, Harlow described him as "devising many plans of future operation, which are no sooner arranged than they are abandoned. . . . In this regard his mind was radically changed, so decidedly that his friends and acquaintances said he was no longer Gage."

At the end of the nineteenth century, Leonardo Bianchi removed both frontal lobes from dogs and noted that they no longer showed affection for people and no longer groomed, but other changes in conative behavior may be difficult to detect in dogs. Some late-nineteenth-century and early-twentieth-century investigators thought that injury to the prefrontal lobes did not cause behavioral changes and claimed that the frontal lobes are a "silent" area. Others, however, described many specific behavioral disorders, such as a loss of speech, and changes of mood such as inappropriate jocularity and aggression, but a change in conation was not well appreciated until Karl Kleist reported in 1934 that many of the soldiers who suffered frontal lobe injury in the First World War were apathetic, with a loss of drive and initiative (abulia). It was, however, A.R. Luria who recognized that abulia, or what he called a *loss of goal-oriented behavior*, was a major factor in the disability associated with frontal lobe injuries.

Although Phineas Gage and the patients reported by Kleist had penetrating wounds of the frontal lobes, abulia can also be caused by closed-head injuries. In the clinic we often see patients who have closed-head trauma after serious automobile accidents and subsequently are unable to resume work. Because they are not weak, numb, blind, or language impaired, people often think that they are merely malingering in order to receive compensation. These people, however, may have suffered serious injury to their frontal lobes or to the fibers that enter and exist them. Their problem is not a desire for compensation but rather abulia, a deficit in goal-oriented behavior. In general, these patients, like Phineas Gage cannot follow through on long-term plans. However, when a biological drive state such as hunger develops, people with abulia from frontal lobe injuries who are passive most of the time, become active. They work to satisfy their immediate basic needs, but they do little to make certain that in the future their needs and their families' needs will be met. When their immediate needs are not met, they easily become frustrated and angry.

Wally Nauta, a Dutch neuroanatomist who worked at MIT, wrote an important paper in 1971 attempting to explain why patients with frontal lobe injuries have trouble with goal-oriented behavior and with self-initiated activities. He noted that information from the outside world is first transmitted to the primary sensory areas in the temporal (auditory), anterior parietal (touch), and occipital (vision) lobes. These primary sensory areas send the information they receive and analyze to their own sensory association areas (see Fig. 4–4). For example, the primary visual cortex, which receives sensory information from the retina, sends it to visual association areas. The visual association cortices analyze this information to determine the shape, color, and movement of whatever is being observed. All these sensory association areas send information to multimodal or synthesizing areas of the temporal and parietal lobes (see Fig. 4–4). These multimodal areas have rich neuronal networks that store memories of the meaning of stimuli and the strategies for solving problems. In people with frontal lobe damage from trauma or disease, these sensory-cognitive systems are usually working, and because they are working, these people are aware of their environment and have retained everyday knowledge. To utilize this knowledge to achieve goals, however, one needs motivation. Knowledge together with motivation leads to goal-oriented behavior.

Motivations or biological drives are present in humans and in more primitive animals such reptiles. These biological drives are mediated by the limbic system and the hypothalamus (Fig. 9–1). Unlike the temporal, occipital, and parietal cortices, which monitor the outside world, the hypothalamus and limbic system monitor the condition of the body. For example, when the blood sugar level becomes

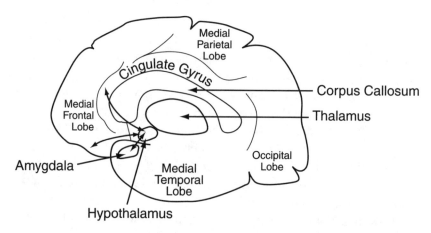

Figure 9–1. Diagram of a midsagittal (cut from front to back) section of the human brain demonstrating the hypothalamus, which monitors body functions. The hypothalamus has reciprocal connections with the frontal lobes and portions of the limbic system, including the cingulate gyrus and the amygdala.

too low, the animal gets hungry and searches for and eats food. When the blood salt level become too high, the animal becomes thirsty and searches for and drinks water.

Patients with frontal lobe injuries have an intact hypothalamus and limbic system, areas that mediate biological drives (e.g., thirst and hunger) and emotions (e.g., fear and anger). Therefore, when they develop a need, they attempt to satisfy it. The hypothalamus and limbic system (which includes the cingulate gyrus and amygdala) send a large number of projections to the frontal lobes (Fig. 9–1). The posterior (temporal-parietal) multimodal sensory areas also send large numbers of projections to the frontal lobes. According to Wally Nauta, the frontal lobe networks fuse biological drives and impulses with the knowledge of how to satisfy them. This fusion leads to the development of goal-oriented behavior, or conation. The frontal lobes project to the motor systems, enabling motivational states to initiate overt behavior.

People with intact frontal lobes are also able to resist immediate biological drives in order to satisfy long-term goals, but when the frontal lobes are damaged, the motivation to reach these goals is lost, although the biological drives and cognitive knowledge remain intact. A farmer we examined had suffered a frontal lobe injury in a car accident. When he became hungry, he wanted food immediately. If he did not get food, he became abusive toward his wife. He also knew that if he wanted food in the winter he would have to plow and plant in the spring, but instead he sat at home and watched television.

The ability to pursue long-term goals and to suppress biological drives is one of the major factors underlying success in any profession. Whereas knowledge, or cognition, is easy to measure, conation is not. One of the most difficult jobs I've ever had was being a member of the medical school's admissions committee. Committee members typically use four criteria to judge applicants: college grades, scores on the Medical College Aptitude Tests (MCATs), extracurricular activities or special talents, and student performance during the interview. Almost every applicant I interviewed had a nearly perfect grade point average (3.8 to 4.0) and performed well on the MCATs. It seemed to me that a more important factor for success in medicine or other careers is the capacity for goal-oriented behavior. Because the frontal lobes are the critical part of the brain for this function, I (colloquially) call this capacity for goal-oriented behavior *frontal intelligence*. Will the students/physicians be willing to stay up all night to take care of a critically ill patient? Will selfish goals be their main source of motivation or will they work for the benefit of their patients and community? I found my work on the admissions committee difficult because I was unsure of how to judge frontal intelligence.

It is unclear if frontal intelligence is learned or biologically endowed. Although intellectual (e.g., language and math) intelligence is partly endowed, keeping children in enriched environments helps develop this intelligence. If frontal intelligence is learned, how do we foster it? When our children were young, my wife and I had a disagreement that, to my mind, has never been resolved. She is a speech pathologist and works with children who have language (reading and speech) disabilities. She believes in operant techniques. Thus, for example, when a child performs well, she or he is rewarded. Because she has used this operant technique at school and has found that it succeeds in changing or promoting certain behaviors, she also wanted to use it at home with our children. I was against the extensive use of this technique because I was concerned about fostering frontal intelligence.

It is unclear how frontal intelligence develops. We know that learning causes the brain to change (plasticity) and that learning can take place throughout life, but certain skills are best learned during certain stages of development. A child who moves to the United States before puberty will have little if any foreign accent, but for one who arrives after age 16, there is a high probability that a foreign accent will be permanent. Henry Kissinger is a good example of this principle. If a child is blind because of corneal clouding and remains blind for several years, when visual acuity is restored with a corneal transplant, the child may still never have useful vision. These observations suggest that children have to learn certain things before they reach critical ages. The frontal lobes are one of the last areas of the brain to mature and may not be fully mature until the person reaches the twenties. This may be why teenagers get into so much trouble. Their increase in sex hormone production creates new, strong drives with a desire for immediate gratification, but with immature frontal lobes they have poor conation. These biological drives and the desires they engender, rather than long-term goals, often control the teenager's behavior. Because children often do not have good conation, educators and parents often successfully use operant techniques to control behavior.

Operant techniques, or behaviorism, were made famous by the Harvard psychologist B.F. Skinner. I first learned about behaviorism when I was in college. Although I was a chemistry major, I took an introductory course in psychology. At the University of Virginia in 1958, the Department of Psychology was strongly influenced by behaviorism and the works of Skinner. Skinner thought that in order to modify behavior, it is necessary to reinforce desired behaviors and avoid reinforcing behaviors to be terminated. We were required to read several books by Skinner, including *Walden Two* and *Of Human Science and Behavior*. These books presented his theories of behaviorism and how the use of operant conditioning principles may make the world a better place. I thought these books were oversimplified and did not deal with several important behavioral issues. After reading them, I asked my psychology professor, "What about the brain?" He replied, "In order to understand behavior, you do not need to know anything about the brain." I also asked, "Based on behavior principles, how do we decide what we should do in the future?" He said, "Your decisions will be based upon how you were rewarded in the past." I was not happy with either of these answers, and based in part, on this class, I decided that I might want to study the brain.

Shortly after joining the faculty at the University of Florida College of Medicine, I learned that B.F. Skinner was coming to Gainesville to give a lecture and I decided to attend. He gave one of the most depressing lectures I have ever heard, stating that we humans are doomed because we can learn only by behaving. When a behavior is reinforced we perform it again, but if it is not reinforced we will be less likely to perform it again, and eventually the behavior will be extinguished. According to Skinner, there is no hope of avoiding a thermonuclear war because the behaviors that would unleash this disaster could not be extinguished until after the behavior became manifest. When listening to this lecture, I thought it was unfortunate that Skinner had not learned more about the brain and how it controls behavior. If he had learned about frontal lobe functions, he would have known that the frontal lobe systems mediate goal-oriented behavior, and this behavior predicats current behavior based on future outcomes. People with intact conative (frontal) systems may not start a thermonuclear war because their knowledge of the outcome may constrain behavior (as it so far has). This is one example of why the development of conative systems is critical, and one possible consequence of using operant techniques excessively in children may be the failure to develop frontal intelligence. To illustrate how these operant techniques may impede conative control systems, consider the story of Solly, the Jewish tailor.

In 1939, Solly left Poland with his family because of Hitler, came to the United States and opened a little shop in a suburb of Indianapolis. Unfortunately, unknown to him, this suburb had a very strong pro-Nazi German-American Association and was virulently anti-Semitic. The members of this Association hoped that his business would fail and that Solly would leave town for New York, where most Jews lived, but because Solly was an excellent tailor and most of the townspeople were not anti-Semitic, his business thrived. The association ordered their youth organization, modeled after Hitler's, to demonstrate outside the tailor's shop. When he looked out of his shop window one summer morning, Solly saw ten teenage boys marching in front of it carrying terrible signs and yelling horrible words: "JEW-BASTARD LEAVE TOWN." "NO HOME FOR KIKES." "CHRIST KILLER."

After looking at the signs for a few minutes, Solly went to his cash register. He took out ten $5 bills, walked outside, and handed one bill to each of boy, saying, "Good job." When the boys returned

to the German-American Association clubhouse, their leader asked
how it went. The oldest boy replied, "Fine, but after we marched
around for a while, that crazy old Jew came out and gave each of us
$5." The leader said, "You and your friends need to march around
each day until that kike leaves town."

The next day, the boys took their signs and again marched outside of the tailor's shop. This time Solly took out ten $1 bills and
gave one to each boy. The following day he gave them 50 cents and
the day after that 25 cents. He continued to reduce the payment
until he gave each boy just a nickel. The next day, the boys did not
march. When the leader of the association saw them sitting around
the clubhouse, he asked, "Why aren't you harassing that kike?" The
oldest boy said, "Hell, it's not worth marching around a few hours
for only a nickel."

Although in this story an operant technique did reduce goal-
oriented behavior, it remains unclear if the extensive use of this
behavior modification system with children inhibits the development of frontal intelligence. More research is needed.

Akinesia: Inability to Move

Abulia can become so severe that even in the absence of weakness,
some patients are unwilling but not unable to move. Their major
problem appears to be an inability to get started by themselves. This
condition is called *akinesia* (*a* = without; *kinesia* = movement). One
of the most dramatic cases of akinesia I have ever seen was that of
Thomas Taylor, a 58-year-old Baptist minister from Deland, Florida.
First, Mr. Taylor developed abulia, but as his disease progressed he
became akinetic. His family brought him to see me in 1971 because
all he did every day after his family got him out of bed was to sit on
the couch. Formerly, when sitting there he turned on the television,
but eventually even this action stopped. Although he had once loved
to talk, now he talked only when someone asked him a question.
When he responded, he usually gave a one-word answer. Two or
three years before seeing me he had been a meticulous, independent, and active man, but by 1971, according to his wife, he did not
even get up to go to the bathroom and often urinated in his pants.
He bathed, shaved, and changed his clothing only when his wife
strongly encouraged him.

I asked his wife how this condition began. She said that her husband had been a hard-working man. Although the members of the church wanted to pay him, he thought it was wrong for a preacher to be paid—a conflict of interest—so he continued working, drilling wells for water, except when someone needed help or on Sundays. The first symptom his wife noticed was that he started being late for appointments. He usually gave a new sermon each week, but then he started repeating some of his sermons. In the last month he preached, he gave the same sermon three Sundays in a row.

While Mr. Taylor listened to his wife give me this history, he was shaking his head. I asked him if her story was wrong and he said, "No, it is correct." When I asked why he gave the same sermon repeatedly, he replied, "If they are dumb enough to stay and listen to the same sermon, they deserve what they get." On hearing these words, a few tears came to his wife's eyes. "Dr. Heilman you cannot believe how much this man has changed. Three or four years ago, I could never imagine him saying anything like that."

On neurological examination, Mr. Taylor showed many signs of frontal-subcortical dysfunction. Some frontal-subcortical behaviors are primitive reflexes that one sees in the infant, such as a hand grasp, a sucking response, and rooting. Normally, as the infant's frontal lobe matures, these reflexes are inhibited, but with damage to the frontal lobe they might reappear. When Mr. Taylor attempted to stand, he had a tendency to fall backward (*retropulse*). When I held him and had him walk he took small steps, another sign of frontal lobe dysfunction. The history of slowly progressive frontal lobe dysfunction suggested one of four conditions: a tumor, a chronic infection, a degenerative disease, or hydrocephalus. In 1971 there were no CT or MRI scans. Instead we obtained an arteriogram, injecting dye into the arteries that supply the brain with blood. This revealed that Mr. Taylor had a tumor pressing on the middle part of both the right and left frontal lobes. We described this finding to him and his wife and recommended that the neurosurgeons remove the tumor. Fortunately, it was a meningioma, a benign tumor of the membranes that cover the brain, and the neurosurgeons were able to remove it completely. I saw Mr. Taylor once at a follow-up visit, and he showed dramatic improvement. He was not preaching but was teaching at Sunday school, caring for himself, and making plans to start work again.

The type of akinesia that Mr. Taylor demonstrated, in which a person remains inactive unless externally prompted, is often associated with bilateral medial frontal lobe lesions (Fig. 9–2). This area of the frontal lobes appears to contain the person's "starting engine," and when this engine fails, as it did in Mr. Taylor, in order to start an activity the person needs to be prompted by someone else. This area of the frontal lobe sends a large number of projections to the motor system, and it is important in activating the motor neurons and hence behavior.

In addition to the anterior and medial portions of the frontal lobes, other regions of the brain that are important in activating the motor cortex. Deep in each hemisphere lie structures called the *basal ganglia* (Fig. 9–3), which receive information from the cortex and send it by an indirect route through the thalamus and back to the cortex. The exact functions of these cortical–basal ganglia–thalamic–cortical circuits are still unknown, but we do know that when they are not working properly, in conditions such as Parkinson's disease, patients have akinesia, or trouble moving. Many people think that patients with Parkinson's disease have trouble moving because they are stiff. While it is true that they are stiff, it is not stiffness that is causing their problem in initiating movements. Their problem is that they cannot will themselves to move, though an external stimulus can help them initiate activity. Before successful drug treatments for Parkinson's disease were available, many patients were

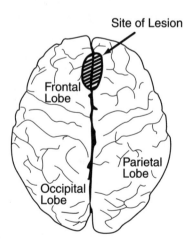

Figure 9–2. Dorsal view of the brain demonstrating a lesion of the medial frontal lobes found in Mr. Taylor, the patient with akinesia (inertia).

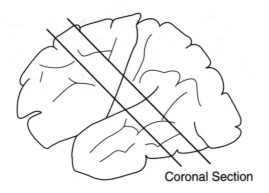

Coronal Section

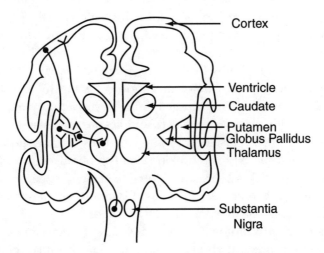

Figure 9–3. A coronal section is a cut through the brain from the top to bottom. This section allows one to see what is under the cortex. This diagram of a coronal section through the human cerebral hemispheres demonstrates the cortex, the basal ganglia (putamen, globus pallidus, caudate, substantia nigra), the ventricles (which contain spinal fluid), the thalamus, and the connections between these areas.

unable to get out of their bed or chair for months or years unless someone helped them. Yet in several reports of fires at nursing homes, these apparently immobile patients were often among the first to leave the burning building. Although in the absence of a relevant stimulus the frontal lobe–basal ganglia systems are important for activating the motor system, the posteriorly located sensory and sensory association systems can also access and activate the motor systems. Disorders of the basal ganglia such as Parkinson's disease and frontal lobe injury cause failures of self-initiation, but sensory stimuli such as seeing a fire, feeling the heat, or smelling the smoke directly activate the motor systems even when the frontal–basal ganglia systems are impaired.

IMPERSISTENCE

Mr. Taylor, the Baptist minister with abulia and akinesia, had a third sign of defective conation. As part of my examination, I wanted to see if Mr. Taylor's sensation was normal. I tested proprioception by asking him if he could feel me moving his big toe. I said, "Mr. Taylor, I want you to close your eyes until I tell you to open them. I am going to move your big toe either up or down. After I have moved it, you tell me which way I moved it." I watched as Mr. Taylor closed his eyes; then I looked down and moved his big toe up. He said, "Up." But when I looked up at him, his eyes were open. I said to him again, "Please close your eyes and keep them closed until I tell you to open them." As soon as I touched his big toe, however, he again opened his eyes. Eventually, I had to blindfold him. Mr. Taylor's inability to keep his eyes closed is called *impersistence*. I also tested his ability to persist in keeping his mouth open; he was unable to keep it open for more than a few seconds.

Patients with motor impersistence may also have impersistence when performing other activities. Mrs. Taylor told me that she thought one of the reasons her husband gave the same sermon more than once was that when he tried to write a new sermon, he worked on it for only a few minutes and then quit. She was describing a form of cognitive impersistence.

Impersistence is also a failure of the "when" system. Mr. Taylor closed his eyes because I told him to do so. My command was an external stimulus. In the absence of repeated external stimuli such as repeated commands, however, he could not continue this motor activity. Andy Kertesz, at the University of Western Ontario, demonstrated that people with impersistence most often have damage to the frontal circuits.

ENVIRONMENTAL DEPENDENCY

Although it is difficult for patients with frontal lobe disease or injury to initiate behaviors themselves, they will often become active when someone else encourages them to act. The behavior of these patients appears to be entirely controlled by the external world. During psychological testing of Mr. Taylor, I put a pen and paper on a table in front of him (so that he could copy intersecting pentagons), but before I showed him the picture I wanted him to copy or gave him any instructions, he picked up the pen and started writing his name. François Lhermitte, described many patients with similar behaviors. One patient was a nurse with frontal lobe dysfunction. When he put a syringe with needle on a table, she gave him an injection. Lehrmitte called this form of environmental dependency *utilization behavior.*

There are other methods of testing patients for environmental dependency. In performing an examination, a neurologist will tell the patient to keep his or her hand open while the neurologist slides the index and middle fingers down the patients' palm. Without instructions to close their hand or to grasp the examiner's fingers, some patients with injury to the frontal lobes or subcortical structures will often hold or even gently squeeze the neurologist's fingers. I often say to patients, "Please do not hold my hand," but after a few seconds, they will hold my hand again. Sometimes, if this grasp reflex is strong, the examiner does not even have to touch the patient's hand. Merely seeing the examiner's hand, especially when it is moving, will cause the patient to reach for it and attempt to hold it. The patient's hands are not the only body part that can inappropriately approach the examiner or other stimuli. Sometimes touching these patients' lips or cheeks will cause them to move their head and mouth so that they appear to want to place the examiner's hand in their mouth. This is called the *rooting reflex.* These same primitive reflexes can be observed in infants, and it is thought that they are important for feeding and holding on to the mother. Like these patients, infants do not have fully functioning frontal lobes. Many of these approach and environmentally dependent behaviors are seen in patients with abulia.

Derek Denny-Brown suggested that as the brain develops, the organism learns specific adaptive strategies to use with specific stimuli. Most of this cognitive knowledge is stored in the temporal and parietal lobes. Normally, when a person confronts an environmental stimulus, the way he or she deals with it should depend on a learned strategy. According to Denny-Brown, the development of the frontal lobes allows a person to avoid responding automatically to a stimulus (environmental dependency) and instead allows the learned strategy to dictate behavior. In Denny-Brown's view, the frontal lobes mediate avoidance behaviors and the temporal-parietal lobes mediate approach behaviors. With injury to the frontal lobes, there is a propensity both to respond inappropriately to stimuli and to have environmental stimuli, rather than long-term goals, control behavior. The frontal lobes are one of the last parts of the brain to mature. That is why young children often act when they know they should not have acted. The game "Simon Says" is a good test of frontal lobe function in children. In this game, the call to action is the phrase, "Simon says." But children will often follow commands not preceded by this term.

A.R. Luria devised a simple bedside test of Denny-Brown's hypothesis. The examiner tells the patient to make a fist with one hand, and when the examiner holds up one finger, the patient is instructed to hold up two fingers. When the examiner holds up two fingers, the patient is to hold up one finger. After the patient has learned these two simple rules, the examiner usually performs ten trials randomly, showing the patient either one or two fingers. Even normal subjects can sometimes make errors, but patients with impaired frontal lobe function will often first hold up the same number of fingers as the examiner and then make the appropriate correction. In another test of environmental dependancy, we have patients put their hands on their lap. We then tell them that when we touch their left hand, they are to raise the right hand, and when we touch their right hand, they are to raise the left hand. Patients with frontal lobe dysfunction often raise first the hand that was touched and then the other hand. When these patients are questioned about the instructions or correct their errors, it is apparent that they know the cognitive strategy. These patients' test performance supports Denny-Brown's hypothesis that with frontal lobe injury it is the stimulus rather than the cognitive goal that controls behavior.

RIGHT–LEFT ASYMMETRIES
OF CONATION OR INTENTION

Although defective response inhibition (a form of environmental dependency) is most frequently associated with bilateral injuries to the frontal lobe circuits, milder symptoms are associated with injuries to the right hemisphere's frontal lobe alone. Similarly, most severe cases of abulia and akinesia also result from injuries to both sides of the dorsolateral or medial frontal lobes, but milder forms of abulia and akinesia are also more likely to be associated with right than left hemisphere injuries. Andy Kertesz reported that damage to both hemispheres can cause the most severe impersistence, but when the injury is restricted to one hemisphere, impersistence is more commonly associated with right than with left hemisphere injury.

In the past 25 years, many people have theorized about the duality of the right and left hemispheres. For example, the left hemisphere has been called the *verbal* hemisphere and the right the *spatial* hemisphere. Others call the left hemisphere the *propositional* hemisphere and the right the *emotional* hemisphere. Although many theorists have warned us about these simple dichotomies, Marcel Kinsbourne suggested that it is fortunate that humans, who love dichotomies, do have two hemispheres. Based on the observation that akinesia, impersistence, and defective response inhibition are more frequently associated with right than with left hemisphere damage, perhaps I will join the dichotomists by suggesting that whereas the left hemisphere is dominant for mediating "how" activities, including how to perform learned skilled movements, how to speak and understand, and how to read and write, the right hemisphere mediates "when" decisions including when to move or act, when to persist at an action, and when not to act. Unfortunately, we still do not fully understand the structural basis for these asymmetries, but "when" decisions are based on goals, and goals, as Wally Nauta suggested, are related to biological drives. Biological drives are mediated by portions of the limbic system, and Albert Galaburda demonstrated in human brains that the limbic system has more connections with the right than with the left hemisphere.

SUMMARY

Cognitive systems such as language (speech, reading, writing), spatial skills, and motor skills provide the knowledge of how to interact and operate within the environment, but they do not provide the knowledge of when to interact. There are three intentional, or "when," decisions a normal person must make: when to act, when to continue acting or persist, and when not to act. The frontal lobes, especially on the right, play a critical role in these decisions. The ability to carry out goal-oriented behavior requires both cognitive knowledge (stored primarily in the temporal and parietal lobes) and motivation or biological drives. Biological drives such as thirst and hunger, as well as emotions such as anger and fear, are mediated by the limbic system, which includes the hypothalamus and amygdala. The frontal lobe fuses these biological drives with the knowledge of how to satisfy them. Through the frontal lobes' connections to the motor system, this fused knowledge leads to goal-oriented behaviors.

Selected Readings

Damasio, A.R. (1994) *Descartes' Error: Emotion, reason and the human brain*, G.P. Putnam's Sons, New York.

Damasio, A.R. Andeson, S.W. (1993) The frontal lobes. In *Clinical Neuropsychology*. (Ed.) Heilman, K.M., and Valenstein, E., Oxford University Press, New York, pp. 409–460.

Levin, H.S., Eisenberg, H.M., Benton, A.L. (Eds.). (1991) *Frontal lobe function and dysfunction*, Oxford University Press, New York.

Nauta, W.S., (1971) The problem with the frontal lobe: a Reinterpretation. Psychiatr. Res. 8:167–187.

Stuss, D.T., Benson D.F. (1986) *The frontal lobes*, Raven Press, New York.

INDEX